C0-AZO-143

THE BRAIN GAME

DOROTHY D. CORRIGAN

THE BRAIN GAME

Exploring and Activating Your Body's Most Creative Organ

Beaufort Books, Inc.
New York / Toronto

Library of Congress Cataloging in Publication Data

Corrigan, Dorothy D.
The brain game.

1. Brain. 2. Intellect. I. Title.
QP376.C66 153 81-6131
ISBN O-8253-0054-1 AACR2

Published in the United States by Beaufort Books, Inc., New York.
Published simultaneously in Canada by General Publishing Co. Limited

Printed in the United States of America First Edition
10 9 8 7 6 5 4 3 2 1

Designer: Ellen LoGiudice

THE BRAIN GAME

Contents

Introduction • 9

1 • The Amazing Brain • 11

2 • A Look Under the Skull • 37

3 • The Brain in Action • 65

4 • Memory, Mentalists, and Mnemonics • 87

5 • Head in the Right Direction • 106

6 • The Expanding Brain • 129

Index • 140

Introduction

Get ready to play the most exciting game in the world: exploring and activating the enormous power of your brain. The unique approach of *The Brain Game* reveals how to use brain power through understanding the structure and physical form of the brain itself.

First, you will discover that the greatest piece of the universe is right inside your head. Second, you will see how your brain works and how each part functions. Third, you will see your brain in action, using language, images, experiences, and environment. Fourth, you will use your new awareness for effective memory and recall, as well as motivation, learning, and thought control. Fifth, you will open a door to new dimensions of thinking and take a giant step toward using your mind in greatly expanded ways.

The Brain Game is more than a book. It will put your gears in action, leading to the development of new thinking skills. New information will be coordinated with daily experiences. To be prepared, have a notebook handy to write in; do the exercises. Above all, have fun while playing the game.

1

The Amazing Brain

The most amazing source of power in the entire universe is right insidc your head.

Computers, adding machines, radar systems—none of these are comparable to the problem-solving capabilities of the human brain.

Consider this: If every person in the world had his own rocket ship, and if all the instructions for take-off, landing, and flight patterns were given through a single master-control tower, this giant communication center would make almost as many connections as those that your brain is called upon to make when you are asleep.

There is a reason for this fantastic mental ability. The

human brain has unlimited power and infinite resources to call upon, while machines can only operate within the boundaries of their design. In short, a machine complements human capability but in no way supplants it.

Part of this limited power can be explained by numbers alone. There are more than 13 billion cells within your head ready to carry messages, record information, remember past experiences, and many other memories. It is the coordinated effort of these cells that think, make decisions, and solve problems. The more you demand of these computing elements, the more they can do, the more shortcuts they will find, and the quicker they will respond.

At This Moment

At this instant your brain is busy. It may seem there is an inactive mass of solid matter within your head, but at every moment during a lifetime the brain is the seething busy control center for the body. Right now neurons are firing electrical signals to receive and react to thousands of messages now bombarding you.

The words you are reading at this moment are entering your brain through impulses in a code of dots and dashes. Here they are sorted, summarized, filed, or discarded. Preferential rating is given those items you may require in the near future. Information filed for permanent storage is reorganized into compartments that match your knowledge, background, and needs. It may be shelved with previous experiences, put with similar data, or activated to create a new file. All input is carefully cross-indexed.

While you are reading and thus recording information from this book, many activities engage your brain to help you comprehend and coordinate all body activities.

As your eyes follow this sentence, your head may go up and down the page; your glance may move back to a previous paragraph. A hand reaches up to anticipate turning a page. Often you pause to reflect on the ideas you are reading about, or you are reminded of something else, and your thoughts wander. Concentration, reflection, association—your brain directs all these activities without conscious commands.

Turn a page ahead, then return to this page. Your fingers were the tool of your brain.

Raise your right hand and spread the fingers far apart. Your brain just sent a message that directed 30 different joints and over 50 muscles to react and do their job. And you hardly had to "think" about it!

Stand up. That change of position took 200 pairs of muscles that needed to adjust and coordinate directions given by your brain.

Keep on reading but "think" about how your brain keeps your body adjusting. When your body gets tired of sitting in the same position, you automatically wiggle, shift weight, or move your shoulders and head slightly to prevent muscles from becoming stiff and sore. You may not notice when you move an arm or cross a leg, but if your wristwatch fell off or something moved beneath your foot, you would probably react immediately.

Underneath your direct attention to this page, are you considering getting something to eat? Are you thinking about walking around the room or making a telephone call? Are you planning what to do tomorrow? If so, you know you are contemplating these ideas and are aware of them in the greater sense, but they are not taking your direct attention. At any moment these ideas may surface and dominate your direct conscious thinking.

Your brain is always deciding what is important to your well-being and what must take priority. This control center is constantly reacting and making decisions to relate you to the environment.

Sudden interruptions, such as the smell of smoke, an exciting television show, or the ringing of the telephone, may take over and push all other thoughts aside.

Many sights and sounds bounce off: the steady drizzle of sleet on the chimney, the whistle of a train in the distance, the movement of a cloud over the sun. Your brain is always alert and responsive to what is—and is not—significant.

Six Amazing Facts About the Brain

There are six major facts about the superiority of the human brain over any other matter in the universe. Each is important to the understanding of brain control and efficiency.

THE AMAZING BRAIN—

1. has unlimited power.
2. is the focal spot for all you know.
3. individually, is unique and different.
4. is part of a universal network.
5. can focus and concentrate.
6. contains infinite potential.

1. The Brain Has Unlimited Power.
Brain power is difficult to visualize. Physiologist W. Grey Walter of Great Britain has figured that to build a replica of the human brain would take a million-and-a-half cubic feet of space.

Picture a football field, including the end zones. Draw imaginary lines to form a box over the field, 26 feet high. The power that could be generated by this large unit would not be capable of free thought or creativity, but would, in a general way, be capable of producing the energy of the human brain. The power of the football field replica can be analyzed, computed, and registered.

THERE IS NO LIMIT TO THE POWER OF THE HUMAN BRAIN.

Each of the 13 billion energy producing cells in the human brain can be integrated, used over and over, and be recombined in new patterns. When you were born, you had all the brain cells or neurons you have now; but a newborn infant does not have many interconnections between them.

As you develop and experience, more paths are connected between cells to create masses of branching patterns and crossroads.

This is where the power starts to multiply in staggering amounts. Thus the same cells that learned and studied and stored the multiplication table might be combined in different channels to recall the pleasure of a recent fishing trip or to consider how the earth originated.

Brain activity is fast. Nerve impulses are constantly flowing like a river throughout your body. Messages travel rapidly, about 3.5 miles a minute or about 450 feet per second. These nerve impulses might be telling you to lower your head to avoid a ceiling beam. Or a nerve impulse could bring the smell of steak cooking and remind you it is time for dinner.

Consider the brain power of Shakuntula Devi. At the age of three she could calculate roots of large numbers, such as the cube root of 140,608 is 52. How she did this no one understood. She had no formal education and lived with her parents in India. Her fame soon spread. In October, 1976, as a young woman, she was giving demonstrations at the American University, Catholic University, and George Mason Community College.

While demonstrating in a classroom in the Department of Electrical Engineering and Computer Science at George Washington University, she beat the calculation speed of a large computer. Then she asked the students to give her any perfect cube of any number. The number 777 was put into the keyboard terminal. Devi had the answer right away—469097433—and the class screamed with delight.

Devi believes her ability is a gift. She does not use commas, saying they confuse her. Devi doesn't like to talk very much about her special powers. She says there is no practical application for them, not wanting to work in mathematics.

Andy Vogt, mathematics professor at Georgetown, said that perhaps Devi possesses some primordial ability that goes back to the origin of life. Arnold Aeltzer, department chairman, said that somehow all that ability was built in her brain.

Power, energy, and speed: These are the greatest resources of the brain. The power generated by the 13 billion cells in your brain is capable of reflecting on the meaning of life or painting an abstract design. The energy can be used as casually as stifling a yawn. The speed can be as crucial as turning the wheel of a car to avoid an accident.

2. *The Brain Is the Focal Spot for All You Know.* You can rub a piece of material with your fingers to get the feel of it, but fingers do not know if the material is soft or rough, thick or thin, dry or wet. The receptor cells of the fingers are probers of the outside world and send messages to the brain. The brain takes in the data, supplements this with the information being received by the receptor cells of the eyes, ears, other senses, and relays it to another department which decodes the messages and checks with stored

picture images and past experiences to decide what your fingers are touching. In the fullest sense of the word, it is the brain that knows.

As the brain is the focal spot for everything you know in a physical way, then it follows that the brain is also the focal spot for *everything* you know and feel, even emotionally. Tears, hate, sorrow, laughter, joy are interpretations made by the brain. The brain is where you enjoy, suffer, dream, and experience.

For example, you see a piece of blueberry pie. The pie on the plate cannot *do* anything to you. But suddenly you might feel happy, sick, or humiliated. It depends on your interpretation of a piece of blueberry pie through emotions connected to a happy memory of picking berries on a picnic, getting sick from overeating, or the time your best friend dropped a piece of bluebery pie in your lap.

Your brain, being the center of the activity for you, can take you anywhere. It can form pictures for you to see, play music for you to hear, or go anywhere in time and space. Musicians can sit in a silent room and hear music they know and with their minds listen to notes, instruments, rhythm, and tune. Actors can rehearse their roles as if watching and listening to a play without saying a word out loud. Golfers are able to practice their swing while sitting in an armchair, or replay, in their mind, a well-played golf game. Everyone has recalled a very pleasant experience step by step, and reluctantly relived a bad scare or a frightening accident.

In all events, the focal spot for everything you know is in

your brain—for outside information gathered by your receptor cells; for emotional reactions such as love and pleasure or pain and sadness; for real and imaginary experiences.

3. Your Brain, Individually, Is Unique.
Your brain is unique. There is not another like it anywhere. Your brain sends waves that can be recorded by a machine. They are as identifiable as fingerprints and change their pattern if you are awake or asleep, if you receive an injury to your body, or if you have a headache. These waves are you—just you—and only you.

Your brain is different from all others because it is your personal memory file, an accumulation of your heredity traits, environmental situations, individual experiences. Although you might think you forget, nothing is forgotten that has been recorded in your mind.

Dr. Wilder Penfield, Director of the Montreal Neurological Institute, started his noted experiments in the 1940s and continued them into the fifties. He started with an amazing discovery during a brain operation. To locate brain damage, he stimulated various parts of an epileptic patient's cortical speech areas.

While the patient was still awake, different areas of his brain were probed and stimulated. He did not feel any pain or discomfort. The probes are often inserted quite deeply, and wires are electrically powered so a current can be passed into the brain. This technique is called ESB, electrical stimulation of the brain. It is used to relieve deep anxiety, immense pain, severe depression, and epileptic seizures.

This procedure triggered memories that the patient had forgotten. He spoke of these recalled events, describing them in vivid detail. It was like he was reliving the original event, watching his past experience much as he might view a replay of a football game. As a different area was stimulated, another set of stored memories was activated. Tests with other patients confirmed these results. One man saw himself at a party in South Africa. A mother saw herself in her kitchen listening to the voice of her son playing in the backyard. She could hear autos, dogs, the laughter of children playing nearby.

Usually the memories are not important. They may be trivial but are always specific. The patient does not lose awareness of the present moment. He knows where he is, can answer questions, and is aware he is remembering. It is as though there are two simultaneous realities; one is in the operating room and one in the past.

There is no one cell or cell cluster where past events are stored. If certain cells are destroyed, other cells take over and do their job. A memory is not contained in one single, special part of the brain but is stored in bits and pieces with a cross reference system. Memory is not a storehouse of facts, data, information, and experiences but a complex arrangement with priorities of importance. The sensory data that has been fed us is still there. Nothing is lost or forgotten. We are living in the past and present at the same time.

Spend a few minutes, right now, and try to remember a happy experience. Replay it in your mind from start to finish. It might be a telephone conversation, a dance, a winning touchdown, a promotion. Think about it again when you are about to fall asleep, or are daydreaming. The more you practice this, the greater your ability will be, under varying circumstances, to remember and develop your brain power.

Everything that happens to you continues to develop your unique brain while expanding your brain capability. Body actions are added to the brain's storehouse. Engrams and neural patterns are recorded, and an actual change takes place in the gray matter of your brain. The stronger or more active the experience, the more change results.

You are your brain. Your brain is you. Here is your inner being, the very center of your existence, the essential core that makes you an individual.

4. Your Brain Is Part of a Universal Network.
Have you ever known the thoughts of another person before he spoke? Have you known who was on the telephone before it stopped ringing? Have you ever felt yourself protected from danger or being guided toward something important for your knowledge? Much of this may be coincidence, but other explanations are possible.

For instance, a mother in California was packing her suitcase when the message arrived that her son, who lived many miles away, needed her. She was getting ready to go to him before the message was delivered; she had dreamed of receiving the message the night before.

Then there was Tom, age ten, who was lost in the Wisconsin woods until he felt he was being led out to safety by an unseen presence. An unknown path, hidden for many years before his birth, was suddenly revealed. He felt someone or something was helping him. His life was saved.

Many people come to Kingdon L. Brown for psychic advice. He is the leader of St. Timothy's Abbey Church in Detroit, Michigan, and a member of many psychic organizations. Brown tells of an unusual psychic experience in his book, *The Power of Psychic Awareness*.

Lee R. a friend of Brown's, was a construction worker whose work was very dangerous. He often thought that if danger was coming his way, he would be warned. One night he dreamed he was on his next assignment in Rochester, New York. Standing on the ground, he dreamed he saw a crane moving a steel beam, it lost control and the beam started to fall on Lee. He awakened screaming.

Lee telephoned Brown, and they decided it was a warning. The next morning Lee was sent to work in Virginia instead of Rochester. Several weeks later, Lee called Brown to tell him there had been an accident at the Rochester site. A beam had fallen, just as Lee dreamed, and injured a workman. He was not killed or hurt severely because he heard a voice that sounded like Lee's telling him to watch out because a beam was falling.

Joseph Murphy, Fellow of the Andhra Research University of India, possesses four doctorate degrees and has written thirty-six books on psychic events, including

Psychic Perception: The Magic of Extrasensory Power. In this book he describes many psychic experiences; two are especially chilling and eerie.

A physician friend of Murphy's was staying in a Canadian hotel while attending a convention. She went to sleep easily but woke suddenly feeling there was a man in her room. She could see him—tall, nice-looking, and holding a gun. He shot himself and fell down dead on the floor.

She called the night clerk who told her that one week ago a man had committed suicide in that room.

A widow told the author the following experience. Her husband had told her shortly before he died that he had made out a new will leaving all he had to her. No one could find the will and the lawyer said he knew nothing about it. She searched everywhere until one day, while ironing in the kitchen, she heard the voice of her dead husband telling her to read Isaiah: 45. She opened the bible and found the new will, all properly made out.

Many people have experiences they cannot explain or understand, but that support the theory of a source of energy outside of the human view of space and time.

Thomas Alva Edison told of receiving ideas out of the air. He believed that they were available to anyone, and said that if he hadn't been receptive to them, someone else would have been.

Dr. J.B. Rhine, an American psychologist, brought a certain amount of respectability to psychic phenomena and extrasensory perception (ESP). Doing most of his studying of psychic experiences at Duke University, he was a world leader and belonged to academic societies throughout the world. He believed that all of us have access to knowledge and ideas beyond our own experience and memory and that most of us have latent psychic ability.

Ralph Waldo Emerson said there is one mind, common to all humans, and that our bodies are like inlets feeding in and out of a large ocean. He believed that there is a universal network that envelops all human beings in an unknown mysterious way.

The clergy calls it a divine spirit. Parapsychologists name it telepathy, extra-sensory perception, or clairvoyance. Scientists refer to it as a cosmic energy and life force.

This universal spirit of the world is difficult to define in ordinary terms or to describe through the experiences of other people. Each person must examine and ponder the concept for himself.

When you have a problem to solve or a decision to make, how do you find the answer? Where are you searching? Almost invariably, when a person is asked this question, he will reply, "I feel that the answer to my problem exists somewhere. Perhaps it is deep inside me or out in the great void. But I know that the solution is available. If I search long enough, I will find the answer. And the fantastic part is that, when I find the answer, and it is right for me, I know it."

Schubert was only one musician who told of remembering a song that he had not heard before, one that led to a new musical composition. Michelangelo "saw" figures and shapes in solid blocks of stone. Louis Agassiz was trying to decipher the shape left by a fossil fish on a stone and was unsuccessful until he dreamed of the fish and in a vision, half asleep, he saw the fish, got up, and made a drawing. With this guide he could chisel more of the stone and find the fossil as he had dreamed it.

Those who find this life force in nature do not necessarily have visions or exchange thoughts with other persons. What usually happens is a greater awareness of themselves and the world, a feeling of comfort and joy, and a unity with a great source of power and knowledge.

Have you ever felt a power source of help outside of yourself? When you are thinking, where do your thoughts go? Go to sleep tonight with these ideas on your mind and see if you awaken refreshed and revitalized.

5. Your Brain Can Focus and Concentrate.
Night and day, asleep or awake, your brain goes right on thinking about ideas, events, sights and sounds without being directly told to and without conscious attention.

This inability to turn things *off* in your mind assists you to meet a deadline, plan an appointment, prepare for a lengthy trip, or accomplish certain tasks. You may call it worry, but with this focusing reminder set in your brain, the only way to obtain release is to complete the idea or task.

This does not mean a negative attitude of getting something down under pressure and fear. It does mean setting an automatic time clock to accomplish goals. This happens through a positive will to succeed. Often a person wishes he could stop thinking about a future event, or forget a certain unsolved situation. But if it is important to him, his brain will keep working on it.

Focusing gets it done. Concentration gets it done efficiently.

Try a short experiment. For ten seconds, try to concentrate with all your attention on *one* specific subject. It can be an object in front of you such as this book, or a goal that you wish to accomplish today. Did you do it? This is hard to do for longer periods, but with practice and discipline you will be able to keep other subjects and unrelated ideas from creeping into your thoughts and distracting you from your prime target.

Get in the habit of finding two or three minutes when you can relax and try to learn to keep a longer attention span. Then think about a single subject. Play with it. Turn it around in your mind. Develop more thinking and ideas about it.

6. The Human Brain Contains Infinite Potential. Man's brain is like a garden with many varieties of seeds to bloom. During a person's lifetime these potentials have no finite end, but can be stretched to infinity.

Usually potentials are thought of as talents and abilities, hidden assets to be developed. Children may show a leaning early in life toward music, art, or mechanics. But potential means much more. It holds the promise of what can come into existence—if nurtured and developed, intensified and expanded.

Some Obvious Potentials Within Everyone

All of the senses can be more fully developed by everyone. Smell, for example, is waiting inside each brain for anyone who wishes to become more proficient at identifying odors. Sensitivity of sight, touch, taste, and hearing can be increased. A greater awareness of the world around us is waiting inside each brain. More responsiveness to our feelings and physical needs is part of our brain potential. An awakening feeling toward our own body can be activated. The brain has a large potential for healing itself, and for making necessary adjustments. Although never be used by most people, this ability is available when needed.

Life was almost over for Thomas Bay Whitman, of North Park, Illinois. In March, 1959, his car went out of control and flipped over several times. He had serious head injuries, was in a coma for ten weeks, and for three months the right side of his body was paralyzed. Eight brain operations and extensive therapy put his brain in working shape again until he was able to sit in a wheelchair. He was dependent on someone else for everything.

One day the doctor said that if Whitman could get out of the chair by himself, he could go home. It was a long agonizing struggle, but he finally succeeded. He went to his mother's house, and there he drew upon his brain's resources to learn how to feed himself, talk, walk, write, and take care of his own needs. He then went back to school to begin a new profession. Soon Whitman was independent and felt his mind was sharper than ever.

Stroke victims often need extensive therapy to retrain their brains to perform tasks easily done before. Whichever hemisphere the stroke was in can affect the other side of the body, and the victim is sometimes speechless, paralyzed, experiences weakness in the limbs, and has sight problems. But the problem is not in the body; it is in the brain. Repeated practice of sending messages from the brain to the affected area takes time and patience, but the brain has great recuperative powers.

Hypnotism can be very successful when used for nervous disorders or relief from pain during an operation. The hypnotist is not a magician; he makes suggestions that a person is able to follow by opening up his potential; the ability, in this case, to enter a trance-like state. Thus a person could use this hypnotic ability to go to sleep, stop pain, and much more—all through his own ability and body control.

What is hypnosis? How does it work? No one is quite sure, there is a mysterious element to it. It is an induced state in which a person is highly open to suggestion, suspends his own thinking, and has faith in what the hypnotizer is saying.

Research by members of the American Society of Clinical Hypnosis has dispelled many myths associated with hypnosis. The hypnotized person is not asleep; brain waves are different when one is asleep than when one is hypnotized. Hypnosis does not alter respiration, pulse, and other body functions as sleep does.

Hypnotism *does* alter human awareness. A person can have hallucinations, think he is burning or freezing when the temperature is normal, drink water that the hypnotist says is a cocktail, and become tipsy. A person in a hypnotic trance can have muscles controlled and be told he cannot lower an arm or unclasp hands. The more he struggles to do so, the harder it gets.

Hypnotism is also a good memory aid. Since all memory is recorded in the brain and the person is highly open to suggestions and wants to respond, he can take a look back with insight. A witness to a crime can often recall the event under hypnosis. A person can relive a traumatic experience that had been hidden in his brain.

What is hypnosis good for? It can control eating, drinking, smoking, anxiety, chronic pain like migraine headaches, and phobias. Sexual problems, such as impotence, have been helped. Pain control is one of the most important uses of hypnosis.

When Dr. David Spiegel worked at Massachussetts General Hospital in Boston, he was in the emergency room where a patient with a severed hand was suffering greatly. The patient was about to be operated on, and in that situation pain killers are avoided. Dr. Spiegel asked the patient if he wanted some pain relief. The patient agreed eagerly. Dr. Spiegel put him in a trance and in about five minutes the man said all he could feel was a tingling sensation as if his arm had gone to sleep.

The most promising, dramatic, and useful purpose for hypnosis is in surgery. No drugs need be used in many operations and thus no side effects are experienced.

A hypnotized person can also be given posthypnotic suggestion. After every operation he is part of, Dr. Ronald Katz, anesthesiologist at the University of California at Los Angeles, leans down and whispers to the unconscious patient that everything is fine, so that the patient will wake up with no nausea, and feel happy and relaxed.

Another mysterious force relating to the brain is acupuncture. Agu Pert and his associates at the National Institute of Mental Health are researching acupuncture. They think that certain areas in the thalamus part of the brain secrete endorphins. These are a natural body chemical that work as a pain killer such as morphine. Five major endorphins have been identified. They are all small proteins called peptides and are produced in the spinal cord and brain.

Acupuncture is an analgesic. It reduces pain but not sensation, so it cannot be used for all operations, such as those requiring much muscle relaxation. Often patients are referred for acupuncture treatment when all else has failed. Experiments confirm that acupuncture can relieve physical pain. At the University of Toronto, the Medical School of

Virginia, and the University of Washington, the research teams found it worked in many experiments.

Why Brain Power Is Not Better Used

Experts of mental abilities say that most human beings use little of their brain power. William James said that about 10 percent of the brain is used, and Margaret Mead estimated that about 6 percent is utilized. That means at least 90–94 percent is not developed. There is a vast gap between what is and what could be.

One of the most unusual cases of early development and utilization of brain power is that of Peter Winston. By the age of eighteen months, Peter looked at the spines of encyclopedia and figured out the alphabet. He started with A and went through to vase and Zygo. At the age of two years Peter gravitated toward books of knowledge on chemistry and mathematics. He also learned to tell time. He understood fractions at the age of three.

The most amazing ability that Peter developed was to tell a person what day of the week his birthday would fall on any year, within seconds of hearing the subject's date of birth. He is intrigued with calendars, diaries, and engagement pads, and fascinated by mathematical calculators; he collects clocks, thermometers, and coins. He became intrigued with weights and measures and soon started collecting them.

In August 1963 when he was five years old, he was enrolled at the Sands Point Country Day School, Long

Island, New York, a school for intellectually-gifted children. He held his teachers and principal spellbound with his mathematical ability and his discussions on concepts of love, loneliness, immortality, and the existence of God.

No one knows how Peter does all these things. Instructors, however, have noticed that Peter is completely absorbed in what he is doing. How Peter uses his brain demonstrates the importance of concentration and high motivation.

The Real Secret

You have an amazing brain. Here is a part of you that is always receiving, storing, generating, developing, and responding. So far, scientists have not found any limit to what the healthy brain can accomplish. The real secret, most of them agree, is not the age or the intelligence, but the will, the motivation, and the stimulation that surrounds each individual.

Efficiency and better use of the brain grow with practice, understanding and development.

Read the following aloud every day for one week. If you miss a day start over again.

> I have an amazing brain. My brain has unlimited power; it is the focal spot for everything I know, feel, and do. My brain is unique and distinct. It is part of a universal network. It contains infinite potential.
> I have an amazing brain.

Please do not read the next chapter right away. First, experiment with the full range of your senses. Break the routine of your usual way of perceiving.

Try as many activities as you wish, but do at least five "quickies" and one "thinkie" before proceeding. You will find them fun and easy.

Activities

Quickies

1. Brush your teeth, comb your hair, and wash your face without looking in a mirror. Can you do them successfully?
2. Eat something. Smell each bit of food before putting it in your mouth. Does smelling increase or decrease the taste?
3. Observe an animal, such as a dog or cat, eat its food. Does the nose wrinkle? How does he start to eat? Later, describe it to a friend.
4. Close your eyes. Listen. When you open them try to recall the sounds. Could you hear the furnace or refrigerator? Noises from the street? The creak of the building? Birds singing?
5. Play the Numbers Game. Count by 4's, starting with 1. Try 2-6-10-14-18, etc.
6. Recall what you were thinking about last night before you fell asleep. Were you listening to sounds around

you or rethinking events of the day? Tomorrow try to recall what you think about tonight.

7. Walk around one room and touch all kinds of objects: chairs, curtains, rug, windows, walls. As you feel each object, rub it carefully with your fingers. Close your eyes. Try to figure out how you know what the object is.
8. Think through the following questions: Can you feel the weight of a watch or ring you are wearing? Were you aware of it before? Do you feel the pressure of your foot on the floor? Are you biting your nails? Are you curling your toes or wrinkling your forehead?
9. For one complete minute try not to think about an imaginary large, furry white cat looking at you through a nearby window. Do not look at the window or think about the stiff whiskers of the cat or the enormous green eyes that keep staring through the window pane.
10. Think about one subject for two minutes. It can be an idea, an object, or an experience. Repeat this exercise often.
11. Close your eyes, not thinking of words of images. Try to keep your mind blank for one minute.

Thinkies

1. Try an experiment in extra-sensory perception. Have a friend sit across the room, shuffling a deck of cards. He should then turn one card over at a time, look at it, and put it down. While he is doing this, you write down

what suit you visualize the card to be (clubs, hearts, diamonds, spades). Compare results. Normal probability is about one in five. Out of one hundred trials, if you score over thirty, you show a high ability. If you test 30 percent or over, you might want to call your nearest psychological laboratory and offer your services.

2. Memorize four lines of poetry. Repeat the poem every day for a week. Do you really know it? Then ask yourself, if ten years passed, could you stand up in front of a crowd and repeat it?
3. Next time you attend a talk at school, church, or any meeting, take a pencil and paper and make a check mark every time your mind wanders off from what the speaker is saying. Afterwards review why this happened. Did you start thinking about a related idea? Was the talk boring? Were you disturbed by someone in the audience?
4. Take an armchair trip, visiting a favorite vacation spot. Can you see the buildings? Are trees, water, or hills visible? Do you see them in color or black and white? Enlarge your view by going around the corner or past a bend. Feel the wet sand under your feet, the hot sun on your face, or the chill of snow in your boots. Watch yourself do what you did there—fish, play baseball, canoe, ski.
5. Compare your brain power with that described in two books. Read *The Child Buyer* by John Hersey, a story

about the misuse of the human mind describing a time when the power of the brain can be purchased. Or read *The Billion Dollar Brain* by Len Deighton. This is a super spy story about a massive brain, built to control the world.

2

A Look Under the Skull

Where the Brain Came From

All forms of life evolved from one common ancestry: the single-celled amoeba. These minute organisms floated in warm tropical waters, tossed about by the current and tide.

One day a change took place in an amoeba. It was a mutation—an accident that happened to the reproductive process. This amoeba was different from the others. If the change was a bad one for the amoeba, it would die and not reproduce itself. If the change was beneficial, it would be better adapted to the environment, survive, and reproduce. Each change was very slight, but over millions of years many mutations occurred.

Centuries passed. New types of primitive life forms grew into being. These early forms of life had primitive nerve-nets and rudimentary tissues of nerve cells called ganglion. Without a brain, their actions were involuntary. They could not control their environment.

With the gradual appearance of the fish, a brain and spine developed. The best qualification for survival in the sea was the ability to search and move around to find food and protection for the fish and its offspring. The search brain developed.

Life began to climb out on land. Here the needs for survival and reproduction were different. Those creatures best qualified to live on the land had a sensitive nose. Or, in the language of evolution, those land creatures that developed slight changes or mutations, making them better adapted for land life, were those who could smell. Grubs and insects, roots to eat and grass to chew, and the location of water were readily available. The smell brain grew.

Those who were to be part of the long path toward man started to climb trees. Now the search brain or the smell brain were not so important.

A tree creature needs to be able to look where he is going, to judge distances, and spot the enemy. He must store up visual memories of experience and places where he can find food, and be able to recognize what is edible.

A different kind of vision developed. Binocular vision, with two coordinated eyes, which move together and focus on one object, evolved. Thus it was possible to view distance and see depth, figure out the position and distance of the enemy, and measure the space to the ground for jumping and attacking.

The creature in the tree could watch, study, and plan. More acute senses, such as touch, hearing, and taste, developed. Awareness of color and texture became good assets.

Living in trees, though, had its problems. Creatures were likely to sit a great deal. Large bodies developed that were cumbersome on branches and it was difficult for them to escape in time of danger. The smart ones left the trees and went back to the land.

Now survival demanded new traits, and changes evolved. An upright position raised the eyes from the ground. Those who could remember and use past experiences could plan ahead. It became necessary to plant crops, build shelters, join in groups for mutual protection, outwit other groups—to think!

The most important development in the progress toward man developed. The brain pushed to the front: forward and upward. It grew and grew until it bulged in the forehead. It is this part of the brain that gives man the ability to have memory, thought, language, and creativity. Man *had* to think, and he did.

Going up the scale of evolution and ability, the brain increases in size:

gorilla	450	cubic centimeters
ape man	450–650	cubic centimeters
primitive man	900	cubic centimeters
modern man	1200–1500	cubic centimeters

Man has the largest brain in proportion to his body. While the elephant and whale have bigger brains in actual size, they also have larger bodies. It is the size of man's brain in relationship to his body that gives him superiority.

It has been estimated that man's brain will increase in the future to a capacity of 2,000 cubic centimeters. It might be that man is just an infant on the ladder of evolution, and that most of his development will be in the future.

The growth of the brain in the nine-month period of human embryonic development follows the same manner of growth as the process of evolution that took millions of years to evolve.

The brain grows by layers.

By the seventeenth day, a tube-like structure forms in the human embryo. One end will become the brain, and the other, the spinal cord. By the third month the fetus has completed the first layer of the brain, deep inside the skull. This is the ancient, primitive part concerned with survival and the inner workings of the body.

The parts that enable the brain to make better adaptations to the environment, increase communication among parts of the brain, and make decisions then develop. From the fourth to sixth month the cortex forms. This is the structure that allows humans to reflect and create. The last three months of the embryonic period are for growth.

When the child is born, the brain is still incomplete. The first year it grows rapidly. By the time the child is three years old, the brain is two thirds of the anticipated size. The human baby is the only infant whose brain continues to grow after birth, giving a longer time for development in size and capacity.

It is these three factors—the structure of the brain in layers, the size of the human brain, and the extended period for development during childhood that make humans unique.

A Look Under the Skull

If you could look under the skull, you would see a solid, inactive, drab mass of material the size of a grapefruit, weighing about three pounds. The lumpy surface of the brain looks as wrinkled as an old prune. The overall dull gray color is broken here and there by a pink glow where blood vessels course through the brain.

You would look in vain to see a creative idea spark or an inspiration flash. No apparent movement, such as a heart beating or lungs expanding can be seen. You would not see any sensory nerves; the brain is not able to feel pain.

There's nothing exciting to touch, either. No tingling sensations or throbbing power surge is present in the brain. Somewhat soft and moist, it feels something like a mushroom.

Three protective agents surround the brain. It almost floats in a thick bath. Fluid and very soft tissue act as a cushion and enable you to turn rapidly, stand on your head, and move without injuring the brain. The skull and membranes protect the brain from outside dangers and make it possible to sustain a heavy head blow or a fall. Around all of this is skin to keep in the fluids and to keep out the dirt and germs.

You would notice that the brain is divided into two parts, called the cerebral hemispheres. Just as other parts of the body come in pairs, such as arms, legs, and lungs, the brain is in two sections. One side dominates the *other* side of your body.

Pound your left fist on a table. The impulse creating this action originated in the right half of your brain.

Which hand do you use to write? The message for action comes from the opposite side of your brain. Most people are right handed, showing brain dominance from the left cerebral hemisphere.

Since you can't actually look inside your skull or feel your brain, there are other ways to determine individual brain activities.

Do you want to *listen* to what is going on inside your head? Take a seashell and hold it to your ear. Or, cup your fingers around your ear and listen closely. The sound you hear is blood rushing near your ears. Twenty percent of the blood circulated from the heart goes to the brain.

Here's how you can *feel* the way your brain adjusts to a change in motion.

Stand in the middle of a large room. Spread your arms out wide and spin quickly. If you do this long enough you will become dizzy and lose balance and fall down. Unusual action is taking place in the hearing organ, located in the bony prominence just behind the outer ear. What is happening is that the inner fluids in your ear canals which give you balance, maintain body position, and adjust you to any change in motion, are not reacting correctly. As you spin, the fluid keeps on moving faster with you. When you stop, the fluid keeps on moving, and you are dizzy until the fluid in the canal settles down.

Major Parts of the Brain

The three major sections of the brain itself are the hindbrain, midbrain, and forebrain.

Hindbrain

Feel above your ears at the back of your head. You have located the hindbrain, called the cerebellum, with your thumb.

The cerebellum organizes body movements. Want to pick up a book, tap your foot, nod your head? The cerebellum will take care of it, acting like a secretary to the big upper brain, taking directions to coordinate muscular activities, equilibrium, and balance. The cerebellum takes the orders, works out the details to send to the body's muscles, and also receives signals from the body's muscles.

Midbrain

The midbrain is very small and is located in the center of the head. It is made mainly of nerve path fibers to and from the brain. The midbrain provides many functions for the eye muscles, such as movements of the eyes and the size of the pupils.

Try this exercise of the midbrain: Prick up your ears. This is an ancient talent made possible by the midbrain section. Animals, hunting and hunted upon, used to prick their ears to hear better and be more attentive. Some people can still do this, showing our link to lower animals.

Forebrain

Above the midbrain section are two very interesting parts of the brain, the hypothalamus and the thalamus. The hypothalamus, which is just under the thalamus, about even with the ears, is the thermostat of the body, acting as a valve or indicator of general conditions and body temperature. While tiny, this remarkable organ is the central headquarters for regulating sleep, metabolism, water retention, sexual drive, and appetite. It is the reason you blush when you are embarrassed or flush when you are angry.

Think of these words, with emotion, and your hypothalamus is working—eat, fight, mate, fear, sleep. It is still a primitive part of the brain, and as such deals with primitive emotions such as fear, thirst, and hunger. Two halves in form, it is about the size of a small grape.

The egg-shaped thalamus is about the size of a walnut. It is the reception center for physical sensations, such as pain or temperature. Placed between the cerebral hemispheres, its biggest job is to act as the receiving and sorting center for the upper big brain. The thalamus receives millions of messages from the muscle sensors, and it filters, sorts, discards, taking care of anything that must be dealt with quickly.

Now we come to the big brain: the cerebrum. This is the largest part of your entire brain, taking up 80 percent of the total brain size. It took millions of years to develop. Brain volume has doubled in the last million years. This most recent addition to the brain, the latest development on the evolutionary path, makes man able to enjoy a Renoir, reflect on yesterday's events, and sing a song. The cerebrum makes you a thinking and reasoning human being.

The crowning glory to the brain of man is the outer rind of the cerebrum, called the cerebral cortex, which took several hundred thousand years to develop. Inside the bony skull, the cortex had to be squeezed into the available space; it is wrinkled with many folds and convolutions.

Here is the most civilized part of your being, the place that creates poetry, grasps concepts, envisions the future, and cares about higher emotions such as love, loyalty, and beauty. It is the site of memory, containing billions of memory traces and bits of information. The cerebral cortex is the control center, the site of all man's thinking and planning. The cortex controls the entire being.

The latest research on the two hemispheres of the brain is astonishing and a real breakthrough in understanding how the brain functions. The new information is based on studies of people who have had one hemisphere damaged by disease or accident. When one side is disabled and nonfunctioning, studies of the side which still works can be analyzed.

Neurosurgeon Dr. Paul Bucy, while professor of surgery at Northwestern University and chief of neurosurgery at Wesley Hospital, had removed complete halves of children's brains in order to cure severe mental illness. These children grew up to be normal, acted like average people their own age, and even attended college.

The cerebral cortex of the brain is divided into two parts, separated by fibers called the corpus callosum. In addition to controlling opposite sides of the body, these half-brains have further functions. The left side controls and directs practical and logical thinking, involving words. The right side is able to see images or pictures.

Left Hemisphere	*Right Hemisphere*
Logical	Makes Pictures
Analytical Thinking	Spatial Orientation
Speech Center	Recognizes Faces

Left Hemisphere	*Right Hemisphere*
Orderly	Awareness of Body
Rational	Processes Information Simultaneously
Linear	Musical, Crafts, Arts Ability
Processes Information in Sequence	Depth Perception
Titles and Classifies Images	Makes Dreams
Verbal	Empirical View
	Takes Unrelated Data and Puts Together in New Form

Both hemispheres seem to work in opposite directions, but actually they work in a complementary manner.

While each is a specialist in its functions, potential exists in either side to do the complete job. So, if one side of the brain is not functioning, through an accident, brain damage, or birth defects, the other hemisphere can assume some of the functions of the impaired side. Language and control of body parts are the most difficult functions to assume. The functional change is gradual depending on how much damage has been done to the brain.

We have been taught all of our lives through schooling and jobs to use the left side of our brain. Reading is a linear technique, where we progress from one word to another and come to a logical conclusion. Studying mathematics, chemistry, and science, we build from one thought to another. This is how we have been taught to make decisions. We need to stimulate the right side of the brain in order to put unrelated information into new ideas and to learn to think more empirically.

Activities

To Stimulate Right Hemisphere

1. Close your eyes, and in your mind walk around your house or apartment. Can you visualize the furniture, views from windows, art, or decorative items? What books or magazines do you see?
2. Close your eyes and in your mind walk around where you were brought up as a child. Where is the living room? Can you identify what is in the kitchen? Your parents' room? What does it look like through the window? Can you see the street or backyard?
3. Picture yourself in a favorite place like a museum or a garden you enjoy working in. Walk around, recalling past experiences.
4. Visualize yourself at a specific event that you enjoyed very much. See the surroundings and the environment. Remember the people. What did they wear? How did everyone behave? See yourself walking and talking. What did you discuss? How did you feel?
5. Get in the habit of visualizing past experiences. Can you see the faces of people you recall? Picture yourself in future events. Visualize yourself becoming more aware of your surroundings.
6. Listen to music. What do you "see" as the music fills

the air? Pictorial program music was composed by musicians who had pictures in their minds and from that they created the music. Saint-Saëns wrote *The Carnival of the Animals* to create a different animal with each separate part of the theme. You might want to listen to other composers whose music reflected images they saw: Mussorgsky (*Pictures at an Exhibition*) Stravinsky (*The Rite of Spring*) and Dukas (*The Sorcerer's Apprentice*). It is not necessary to "see" what they saw; just enjoy the music and watch the pictures that flow through your mind.

Doing the above exercises will promote your imagination and intuition, stimulating the right hemisphere of the brain.

The Brain Stem and Spinal Cord

Underneath the brain itself is the brain stem. Feel the lower part of the back of your head where it slopes inward, behind your ears. Here is the brain stem, a column about three inches long, functioning as a channel for tracts of nerves running to and from the brain and spinal cord.

The brain stem has two sections. The upper part is the pons, a bridge of fibers uniting certain portions of the brain. The lower is the medulla, serving as a reflex center with special duties for the involuntary nervous system such as maintaining respiration, heartbeat, blood pressure, swallowing, salivating, sweating, and sneezing.

Through the center of the brain stem runs the reticular

activating system, which coordinates incoming sensations. It alerts the upper parts of the brain to what is important. For example, it explains why a mother is aware of her child crying in the street but does not always hear other street noises.

From the brain stem runs the spinal cord. It is eighteen inches long and ends in the center of the small of the back. This is the pathway from the brain to all parts of the body.

Harmonious Action

Each part of the brain has specific duties, but all parts function together in working out decisions. It is a balance of harmonious action.

The deep, older portions of the brain are busy with basic urges and desires that keep the body seeking food, shelter, sex, and safety. The old brain is constantly saying, "Let's get going. Here is the situation and something must be done about it."

The hypothalamus is likely to add, "I have an emergency that must take top priority."

The thalamus says, "I've sent several messages up recently. Get moving on them."

The cerebrum might answer, "Now you know I am a policy maker and a top executive. I don't like to be hurried. I need time to reflect on the problem. Right now I am contemplating a lovely sunset; the blues and pinks and gold blend in such a beautiful pattern. What was it you wanted?"

Parts working in unison are necessary to your well being. John Pfeiffer, in his book *The Human Brain*, estimates that about 100 million electrical impulses bombard your body every second of your entire lifetime. Out of all these signals and messages, about 100, or one out of a million, impulses reach the upper part of your brain. It is a good arrangement. Low-level sorters and decision makers handle routine, basic needs; otherwise there would be no time for thinking and planning ahead. The development of higher thinking levels enables you to have a special place for evaluating, judging, and decision making.

To find more about your "thinking" right now, do the following exercise.

How to Begin to Think Better

Memorize the following two statements:

1. Forebrain thinking is intelligent and thoughtful.
2. Hindbrain and midbrain thinking is primitive and quick.

The back and lower parts of the brain push us to make quick decisions, and experience intense feelings of anger along with sudden reactions of fear leading to panic. This is necessary in moments of physical danger or emergency, but too often the old brain of survival dominates.

Man's forebrain gives him the power and ability to think things over, to put seemingly unrelated items together to form new images and new ideas. It allows us to envision from a different perspective, to let decisions germinate and ripen.

How can we take advantage of this? Use the forebrain and realize what you are doing.

Take action and start analyzing your thinking to develop more forebrain use. Observe and study conversation, moments when you and others are expressing thoughts and discussing ideas.

Can you remember a time when a discussion hit on a special topic and you reacted strongly? Or when someone made a statement that infuriated you? You spoke out, using heated words and rapid sentences, and you felt carried away. Later you might have realized you didn't argue convincingly or make yourself clear, and you wondered why.

As you become involved in future conversations, watch not only for your own thinking (forebrain) and rash quick reactions (hindbrain and lower brain) but also watch others. Do the persons making the best and most appropriate statements and convincing conclusions lose their temper, becoming red and flushed? Do they listen to anyone else? Who expressed the best and most thoughtful ideas? Is self-control important? Compare thinking and anger. Are they compatible?

When there are several people talking, remain silent and observe your own reactions. How are you responding? Do you want to give quick and easy answers? Are certain points being made for progress? How can you help move the dialogue forward? How do you feel—comfortable? Inferior? Stupid? Secure? What is going on inside your head?

Another important use of forebrain thinking is to prevent yourself from making rash decisions when deep thought and time for reflection are necessary.

The way to do this is to say to yourself something like the following:

> I am not going to solve this problem right away . . . It is complicated . . . I am not going to force myself to find the right answer immediately . . . What I am going to do is analyze the situation, let it set awhile, perhaps sleep on it. I will put it on the back burner, so to speak. I will let it be a thoughtful unconscious pondering, like planting seeds and letting them sprout on their own.

Bill Lear, of Lear jet fame, knows how to do this. A genius at solving problems having to do with radio and television sets, jet planes, and pollution-free automobiles, he says he cannot explain how and why his ideas create themselves. They just come out of his head. He says he deliberately feeds information into his mind and then proceeds to, just as deliberately, forget about it. During an unlikely moment, the answer eventually pops up. While dining at a New York restaurant, the idea on how to design the circuitry for a jet autopilot popped up, and he quickly sketched it on a napkin.

Solutions to problems are not usually a sudden flash or inspiration. Unconsciously, our forebrain has been wrestling with the problem and eventually comes up with the answer.

The Nervous System

Two nervous systems operate in the human body—the automatic and peripheral.

The automatic nervous system keeps right on working at all times below your level of consciousness.

Using the spinal cord with direct routes to the internal organs, it controls digestion, breathing, blood vessels, and circulation. It has the responsibility of conserving the body's resources and preparing your body for strenuous action and emergencies.

The peripheral, or voluntary nervous system, is mainly yours to command.

The system is a two-way path. Sensory nerve cells bring information from the skin, muscles, and sense organs to the spinal cord, brain stem, and brain. Other types of nerve cells—motor nerve cells—take the brain's orders back through the spinal cord to the muscles, fingers, feet, etc. These messages or impulses are bits of information picked up by sensory units and passed on for interpretation.

All impulses are transmitted through nerve cells. One type is the neuron, a minute cell which can be seen through a microscope. Every neuron has three main parts: body, dendrite, and axon. The impulse is received by the dendrite, passed through the cell body, and sent on by the axon. The axon of one neuron comes close to the dendrite of another. The gap between is a synapse. The action is but a chemical/electrical transaction that takes place when one neuron fires an impulse to its neighbor.

The purpose of the entire nervous system is to conduct these electrical impulses.

Impulses move quickly, ranging from two to two hundred miles an hour. The fewer neurons involved, then the shorter the distance to travel, and the more rapidly the messages arrive.

Once you start to respond to a stimulus (something outside the body), your nervous system wishes to take action. A stimulus pushes us into doing something. The action is the response. When we have responded, satisfaction and relaxation are the result.

Many responses are reflex actions, reactions to a situation that occur without consciousness. This is largely involuntary. Simple reflexes are numerous in lower animals as well as in man. Removing your finger from a hot stove, blinking your eyes at a sudden light, jerking your knee when the doctor taps below your knee are all reflex actions. These reflexes are responded to by the spinal cord.

Other reflex actions, not quite so fast, are more complex, but still produce almost automatic reactions. Running from danger, becoming hungry at the sight and smell of food, driving a car by habit, are all examples of this type of reaction. In these cases the action of the body is taken care of anywhere from the spinal cord to the brain stem, or the lower part of the brain.

In both cases, simple reflex and more complex reflexes, a message is reported to the brain. But there is a momentary time lag. That is why you "know" after the action has been taken. Awareness follows.

Actions taking higher decisions and involving thinking go to the brain itself. It might be a decision on how to react to a car careening along the highway, or ways to complain about an injustice. This type of thinking has the longest route to travel, goes to the highest part of the brain, and has the longest reaction time.

Write these three terms across the top of one page. Simple Reflex. Reflex. Thinking. Under each put the following descriptions:

Simple Reflex—rapid action, shortest route, goes to the spinal cord, not controllable.
Reflex—quick action, middle route, goes to lower brain, automatic.
Thinking—longer reaction, longest route, goes to highest brain, controllable.

The Nervous System—Using It More Efficiently

The brain can only react to what it is given. Scientific testing has shown that people in isolation, given only water and basic nourishment but no sensory input, do not behave like themselves. There is a loss of time sense. Sleep becomes their overwhelming need. The brain needs stimulation. Color, texture, images, sounds, and sights are necessary for efficient brain function.

The nervous system wishes to complete the arc of stimulus—response—action. So, get started on what you want to do. Need to prepare for a trip? Get out a suitcase. Want a raise? Ask for an appointment with the boss. Wish to answer a long and involved letter? Write the first sentence. How it will all work out doesn't need to be determined. Once involved, your nervous system will respond, and you will work toward completion and satisfaction.

When you are working on a lengthy project, keep your ideas active in your mind. No one knows this better than writers. A long written assignment, if left for days or weeks, almost requires starting over again. Less warm-up time is needed if the ideas are fresh in your mind. When other activities do take your attention and prevent you from continuing for a period of time on a project, at least give it thought often. Review it during the day. Let it be working for you even while you are not directly working on it.

While the nervous system needs stimulation and activity,

confusion can result if too much information is received, or if interfering sounds prevent you from keeping on the thought-track. Turn off the radio or television. Drop out of the surrounding conversation or overstimulating events around you. Input circuits can only take in so much; when overloaded, the brain makes errors, omitting vital information from the senses and delaying reactions.

Train yourself to be honest and accurate in your observations and uses of the senses. Remember that the nervous system can only react to what it is fed. If the incoming messages are not accurate, the brain cannot respond accurately. Eyes look, and the brain interprets. The ears hear, but the brain listens. The fingers touch, and the brain identifies.

How can we be more accurate? Try the following exercise. Practice remembering places, people, experiences. Close your eyes and in your imagination, walk down the block where you live. Can you see the details? How about the people who live there? Recall their faces, expressions, eye color, hair, skin, clothes, mannerisms.

After a talk session, compare the reactions and views of others with your own.

Check with yourself often by asking yourself, am I getting the message? What is happening in front of me? What are the main points; what is the strategy? When reading, summarize the main thoughts. Read a news article and then deliberately explain it to someone.

Look in the mirror with eyes that you pretend belong to

someone else. What do you see? How would you describe yourself to a stranger, your mother, a friend? Can you be objective?

Continue training to keep input to your nervous system accurate. We tend to see what we want to see, hear what we wish to hear, feel what we desire to feel. Observe. Speculate. Analyze.

Thinking is hard work. A clear head and thoughts must be balanced with periods of rest and detachment. Learn how to relax your thinking. If an arm gets tired throwing a ball, you know when to quit. Or, if you are swimming and your back is tired, muscles won't respond. But when the brain gets tired you get sloppy and undisciplined. Brain fatigue-time is marked by tired, fuzzy thinking.

Try these exercises to relieve tiredness in thinking. They are designed to relax the main parts of the nervous system. If thoughts bubble up in your consciousness, let them float away. Breathe deeply.

1. Fold your arms in front of you. Then raise your wrists to touch your forehead. Hold. Take a deep breath and at the same time raise your arms over your head. Exhale slowly while moving your arms behind your head. Hold. Take another deep breath and return to original position. Exhale slowly. Continue until you feel relaxed.
2. In bed or on the floor, stretch out on your back, closing your eyes. Put your hands under your head. Lift your

head with your hands until your chin touches your chest. Then let your head down flat again, slowly. Next roll your head from side to side, relaxing the mouth, jaw, and facial muscles. Continue until you feel relaxed.

Using The Mind

All the parts of your brain are ready to be used. However, one important factor inhibits this marvelous go mechanism, the feeling of "I can't do it."

Inexperienced parents, overzealous teachers, jealous friends, and misinformed people all give us a negative attitude. Fear of failure adds to a sense of insecurity and feelings of inadequacy. This causes a barrier between the go power of the brain and the fears of the personality.

Try to recall times when you failed in school or at a task. Why did it happen? Was it lack of understanding the assignment or feelings of inferiority? Now remember a time when you had a big success. What was different? Attitude? Basic information? Curiousity? Did you wish to prove to yourself or others you could succeed?

Future success is built on former success. Forget failures.

Remember what a wonderful "go" mechanism you have in your brain. Recall the physical parts and their amazing properties to give you the ability to "do what you want to," and become a continually better-functioning "thinker."

Review the sections in this chapter on brain evolution,

the growth of the human embryo, the structure of the brain and its parts, and how the nervous system operates. Describe what you would see if you could look under the skull and observe the workings of the human brain.

What are you going to do to increase the efficiency of your thinking?

Read through the following activities. Why is each one at the end of this chapter?

Try as many as you wish, but before reading Chapter 3, be sure to do 1, 5, 7, and 12 of the "Quickies," and 2, 4, and 7 of the "Thinkies."

Activities

Quickies

1. Picture yourself with three more eyes. Where would you put them?
2. Describe how the sky looked yesterday.
3. Imagine the world if suddenly earthworms were the size of rattlesnakes. What images do you see?
4. Would you like to be invisible for one day? If people could not see you, how would they detect your presence? List five ways.
5. Do part of a task. Start to make a bed, mow the lawn, or write a letter. Go halfway and stop. How do you feel? Do you want to finish or forget about it?
6. Consider: Does a banana taste differently when you eat

it in hand and peel the skin? How does it taste when you slice it and eat it from a plate? Give reasons.

7. Stop thinking for one minute. Close your eyes. Bring your thoughts out in the air. Picture them resting about 6 inches in front of your forehead. Think of your thoughts blending into a gray foggy mass. Think no words. Concentrate on the gray mass. Try this for two minutes, then three.
8. Try an oriental detachment exercise. Say to yourself over and over, the word "om" for one minute. Do not try for associations, pictures, or ideas.
9. Watch an animal such as a dog or cat. See how he knows his master, sniffs at strange objects, and follows the tracks and the leavings of other animals. Does he hear and look with accuracy?
10. Observe a baby with a new object. Make a list of what he does with it. Look for touch, taste, and developing senses.
11. Play with a word. What does it mean? Say it out loud several times. Use it in different ways. Does the sound of the word have anything to do with its meaning? Try the word in sentences. Use the word five times today.
12. Play with your name. Roll it on your tongue. What kind of a person does it evoke in your mind? Think of nice words to describe the person with your name.

Thinkies

1. Tell two people within one week the following facts:

"The present size and growth of the human brain was reached during the time of Neanderthal man 100,000 years ago. The growth and basic development has hardly changed since then."

2. Find out which eye dominates your vision. Take a piece of paper, tearing a small hole in the center. Hold the paper at arm's length and locate an object across the room. Now bring the paper to your face, slowly, keeping the object in focus and in the center of the hole. The paper will come to the dominant eye.
3. Read *The Sword in the Stone* by T. H. White. The young boy in the story, the future King Arthur, is able to become an ant, bird, or fish through the magic of Merlin. Discover how the boy's thinking changes with each creature he becomes.
4. Read an article, short story, or news story once. Make a mental outline as you go along. Within one day tell it to a friend.
5. When you have an important reason to get up at a certain time in the morning, set your mental alarm clock to awaken five minutes earlier than you have to. Also set your alarm clock for precaution. See if it works and if your control mechanism can wake you on demand the next morning.
6. Memorize the following definitions:
   cerebrum—brain (Latin)
   cerebellum—little brain (L.)
   thalamus—type of room (Greek)

hypothalamus—under the thalamus (G.)
reticular—little net (L.)
efferent or motor fibers—carry outward (L.)
afferent or sensory fibers—carry toward (L.)
cortex—bark (L.)

7. Develop a picture of yourself in a new experience. Picture yourself in new clothes. Practice a new technique on the golf course. Interact with a new group or combination of friends. See yourself walking around in a new image. Can you?

3

The Brain in Action

The brain is constantly in action. Thoughts and ideas flow through it continuously. From the day of birth to the day of death they never stop. Yet, how little we understand what is happening in the core of our center. Even experts differ and many mysteries exist. Let's ''think'' about our thinking.

That's hard to do.

We can take a detached view of a hand. Hold it up; look at it. Rub the skin and nails; feel the bones. Wiggle the fingers. Turn the wrist, then make a fist. Notice the position of the grasping thumb to the fingers. See the veins under the skin. You can get a fairly good idea of your hand and its parts by examining it.

We can't take that kind of a detached view of our thinking. But, by "thinking" about the process we can change it.

Here is one way to get started exploring your thought patterns. It may be frustrating and confusing at first, but practice improves your ability to understand your brain in action.

Sit and ponder for a few minutes. Write, if you wish, some of the thoughts on paper that pass through your mind. Don't try to control your thinking: just let your mind take over. Now, choose a specific subject. Try the hand, for example.

A woman concentrating on her hand might think something like this:

> What a wonderful tool my hand is . . . so flexible. Look at the fingers moving around. Look at that burn from the hot pan I touched yesterday. Stupid, hurts too. Better wear gloves to church tomorrow. I wonder if Bob will be there. He hasn't called for awhile . . . He has good, strong hands. How comforting it is to hold hands with someone you like. I should take better care of my hands, the nails are so funny looking. When I was a little girl I remember how my Aunt Elsie would shame me. I would double my fingers up so you couldn't see my nails, but you always looked anyway. I wonder where you are now . . . You're probably examining hands in heaven. Are there hands in heaven? There's Michelangelo's painting of God with His

long white beard reaching out His hand to give life to Adam. Life, what is it?

The connecting link was hands, but the thought patterns did not flow in a logical, linear manner. They darted to and fro, up and down like a yo-yo, from subject to subject.

Time did not stay in the present. It shuttled back and forth from the present to the past and into the future, from yesterday's burn to abstract thoughts on heaven.

What were the tools or techniques she used to think with?

Words. Language was the key to express her thoughts.

Then, images appeared in her brain. She "saw" her aunt, and visualized being in church. She could see the painting by Michelangelo.

Third, hands were seen as a symbol. Dirty nails were associated with the anxieties of growing up and trying to please adults. Holding hands was a symbol of love. The symbol of an old man with a flowing beard holding his hand out represented God.

We think through three basic techniques: (1) Language. (2) Images. (3) Symbols.

Words describe your thoughts to you. Images flow in front of you. Symbols interpret and move your thoughts to another dimension.

Language

When primates came out of trees and the forebrain developed, civilization progressed. Along with this progress came language. Mankind began self-expression and began growing into a different type of being.

There is logic in this. Brain growth and words developed with each other. Civilization and modern people would not have become what they are today, if they had not evolved language. With language they could think thoughts to themselves, make plans, express hopes, and communicate with others. Sign language, grunts, and gestures, like pointing toward danger, just would not do.

As the forebrain enlarged, words and sentences for speaking and writing became necessary to record and remember. Information could be passed to succeeding generations. Words started with concrete names, like tree, woman, cave. Then expressions were added, like hunger, fear, cold. More abstract concepts developed, such as friendship, sympathy, philosophy, ethics, and theories on death.

The more words you put into your brain, the more your thinking capacity enlarges and is enriched. Life and learning depend on words for reading and writing, talking and listening.

Children from ages six to ten learn about 5,000 words every year. Adults, on the average, learn less than 150 words per year.

Success and high achievement correlate with vocabulary knowledge. Johnson O'Connor, founder of the Human Engineering Laboratories, has examined thousands of people and tabulated the results. High achievers in almost every field scored high in vocabulary use. O'Connor's opinion is that while aptitude tests show the direction people should take, vocabulary tests can determine how far a person will go in his or her career.

Several years ago, studies on the importance of vocabulary knowledge were made by Paul Diederich of Educational Testing Service, which prepares and gives tests for educational institutions. Many tests show that college students who have the highest scores in vocabulary are more successful after leaving school.

Dirk Roberts (not his real name) had always wanted to be a doctor. When he failed the entrance exam for college, he refused to let this stop him. He took several tests of aptitude and word knowledge. He scored low on vocabulary, at the 23 percentile. Doctors usually score about 75 to 77, a high percentile. He used the Johnson O'Connor *Vocabulary Builder*, a group of words listed in order of difficulty. Roberts worked hard on vocabulary building by avidly reading newspapers, magazines, and books. He made a record of every unknown word he came across, looked up all the definitions, and kept reviewing his notes. He said it was like playing a game. He was surprised to find that once he knew a new word, he would come across that word many times. In a year he passed the college entrance exams. He had doubled his vocabulary rating to the 58 percentile. Now he is a doctor and still continues to build his vocabulary.

How can you increase your vocabulary? Do just what

Roberts did: Read everything at hand. Write down all words you come across that you can't define. Maybe you have a vague feeling about the meaning, but can you give an accurate definition? If not, you do not really know it. Play with words. Gather them like flowers to nurture, admire, arrange, and rearrange.

The books of James Joyce are fine examples of wordplay. In his book *Ulysses*, the heroine, Mrs. Bloom, asks her husband the meaning of a word she has come across, "met—him—pike—hoses." He explains it means metempsychosis, the transmigration of souls. This presents a leitmotif, or theme, throughout the novel.

Even Joyce's characters have names that are colorful and rhythmic with hidden meanings: Molly Bloom, Blazes Boylan, Buck Mulligan, and Stephen Dedalus.

Sometimes Joyce gives new meaning to old words and often uses an obscure defintion. Joyce manipulates words so gracefully and with such acumen that the whole book is full of word games such as puns and figures of speech, and bristles with metaphors and similes. Wit, humor, and innovative ambiguities are utilized. Every page is a joy to read, teeming with living language.

As new meanings are needed in the world of language, words change. Old words acquire new definitions. Combinations of old words create different impressions. Consider such words as: supersonic boom, shopping mall, jet stream, drugstore cowboy, checkmate, dramatic irony, subliminal perception. Keep a collection of new word combinations. Make up new ones.

If you have more knowledge of words, you will learn more ideas, express yourself more fluently, make better decisions, and ultimately increase the quality of your life. In short, you will become a better thinker.

Images

Would we be human beings without the ability to see images? Try to imagine life without pictures appearing in your brain. Make a list of how different it would be. As you read through this section, you may want to add to the list. An image can be any of the following:

1. A likeness to or similarity of a person, animal, or thing.
2. A representation of an idea or concept.
3. A reliving of an experience.
4. A form, semblance, appearance.
5. A counterpart or copy.
6. A picture or representation in the mind.
7. Something imagined or conceived by fancy.

Images make it possible for us to read a book and visualize the people and events, or to attend a play, athletic event, or classroom discussion and replay it later, or to plan ahead to see yourself accomplishing a goal.

Alexander Eliot, who was an art editor of *Time*, has a remarkable ability to see images. He wrote *Sight and In-*

sight, a book containing vivid descriptions of paintings, sculpture, and architecture, and his interpretations of them. In 1958 he took his wife and three children to stay in a small Spanish village, but he took no research material or photographs with him. He carried with him images from his past knowledge of art, because from traveling a great deal he had seen much of the world's art and was acquainted with most of the major artists. He could remember many works of art and their impressions on him.

Picasso did the same exercise. He could visualize color. He would walk around the Tuileries and fill himself up with images of green and then go to his studio, see the colors in his mind, and do a green painting.

Visualize some familiar objects that you have known in your life, like the houses or apartments you have lived in. How much detail can you visualize? Do you see the objects in color? Could you write a good description of them?

Sometimes we have preconceived ideas so that when an image appears, the pattern has already been established. We have an image of what a wedding or a bullfight should be like.

Recall some images you have buried in your mind. Sit quietly, eyes closed and see what images you see of the following:

War
White rabbit

School
Hero
Hatred
Beauty and the Beast
Christmas tree
Football
A red rose
Affection

Now go through the words again and try for a different image.

Dreams are another form of images we see. People, places, and experiences flow in front of us as we sleep.

Many scientists are studying dreams, analyzing the pictures the dreamer sees, and theorizing on how dreams relate to the brain.

In 1953, Dr. Nathanial Kleitman observed that sleeping children have rapid eye movements. Their eyes move back and forth, quickly. Dr. William Dement, of Stanford University Medical School, called it REM (rapid eye movement). Sleep laboratories started working with adults who have more complicated dreams and extensive REM. When the REM is occuring, most dreams take place. It is an active time; the whole body is involved. Respiration and heart act in an irregular way, sometimes speeding up as the eyes move faster. The dream may last from ten minutes to an hour, lengthening as the night goes on. Most people dream four to six times a night.

Many reasons are given why we see pictures when we sleep. As a psychological function, the explanations vary from adjusting us to our daily life experiences to escaping from conflicts. But researchers now believe that the neurological role is the most important dream function.

When Dr. Howard Roffwarg, of the University of Texas Health Sciences Center, while monitoring brain waves during REM sleep, noticed electrical activity surging forth from the part of the brain called the pons to the cerebral cortex. He believes that perhaps the brain is trying to make sense out of its electrical signals.

Stanford's Dr. Thomas Anders theorizes that dreams put memory in patterns to help retention and learning. The researchers at the Health Science Center of the University of Texas have a theory that dreams stimulate the brain and develop the nervous system.

While dreams are easily forgotten, all sleep researchers agree that dreams must be important to our well being.

Dr. Carl G. Jung, who formed his own school of psychology in Zurich and was a major force in the psychoanalytic movement, had different ideas on images and dreams. He believed that a person becomes whole when he knows and can accept his unconscious, learning this through dreams and images. He felt that knowing the unconscious is important because it is the guide and adviser to the conscious part of the brain.

Within the unconscious part of a person's psyche is the individual unconscious and the collective unconscious. The later is inherited from our ancestors. The collective unconscious is the culture of mankind with its mythological qualities that go back to primordial images. Their beginnings came with the beginning of the species and are transmitted down by each generation. The part of the brain that retains and transmits the common inheritance of mankind is so old that modern man cannot directly understand these images. Envision some of these ancient images and the myths that surround them, such as snake, sun, moon, solstice, fertility. Jung believed that archaic images are as instinctive to us as migrating is to birds. The brain has its own history and keeps many traces of the stages of its development. We carry with us the memories and history of mankind.

Images are internal, moving, and have a dynamic quality. Symbols are external and static.

Symbols

A symbol is that which suggests to us something other than what it appears to be. What does this mean to us? How can we use this for better thinking?

First, let us recall some symbols we all know: a lion meaning courage, white for purity, red for danger. Flags, numbers, musical notes, business logos, and emblems, are all symbols.

Let us consider some more complicated symbols. The wedding ring is a symbol of commitment. Put in a larger more universal sense it is a symbol of a circle, a symbol of completeness and continuity. The medical profession uses the emblem of the caduceus—two serpents twined around a staff, crowned by two wings. The wand symbolizes power. Snakes denote wisdom. Wings refer to lofty intentions. Both the ring and caduceus have been known for centuries to have been widely used and interpreted.

Now, be ready for a big step in perception. The conscious part of ourselves is mentally awake, alert, and aware. The unconscious is that part of us that is below the threshold of consciousness. We are not conscious of it, nor do we realize how much it influences our behavior and our conscious minds. We meet it in our dreams.

Symbols are the language of the unconscious. Since the unconscious is the unseen adviser and guide to the conscious, the more we understand both, the more we grow and learn and understand. The more we unite our unconscious and conscious, the more we become a complete human being.

Understanding symbols opens up a whole new world to us. J.E. Cirlot, author of *A Dictionary of Symbols*, says that we are symbolizing animals and that at all stages of development of civilization, people have used symbols.

There is a universal quality to symbols. We recognize them. Sometimes we see them without fully understanding their significance. We "know" them intuitively.

Religion and symbols have always been entwined. Church architecture is flooded with symbolic language. The dome of a church stands for the canopy of heaven. Spires point and reach upward. Gothic architecture repeats three doors for faith, hope, and charity. The gutter of a building for carrying off rain water, such as at the Cathedral of Notre Dame, is made in the form of gargoyles. These grotesque, evil-looking monsters with human or animal heads, are symbols of the underworld.

In this century, Le Corbusier designed vertical houses on pillars. His Savoye House in France, designed as a cube, is elevated on pillars. Pillars imply an upward thrust of self-affirmation, have a phallic connotation, and are related to the world axis or eternal stability.

Good poetry is universal and transcends time. It speaks to our unconscious. The poet, Robert Frost, believed that all good poetry said one thing and meant another. His powerfully haunting poem, "Stopping By Woods on a Snowy Evening," is a four stanza poem about a man on the way home who stops to look at the snow and the woods but realizes he must go home to his family. Reading it several times, and letting it sink in, a reader might wonder: Why is it "the darkest evening"? Is there "some mistake"? Why does he have "miles to go" before he sleeps?

This seemingly simple story should be individually interpreted as to what is being revealed, and what is being symbolically said. Dark, mistake, and sleep could be symbols of death. Or, a man who is lonely and tired yearns for silence but must keep going because he has made promises.

The artist is spokesman for his time. Modern artists

appeal to the conscious and unconscious of us all. Many artists express themselves unconsciously; that is the only way their work can be accepted and admired. Art is full of symbols. Look at a Dali painting. See the limp watches draped on an eerie landscape. Look at Paul Klee's colorful circles and circles. Bull's-eyes and colorful spheres abound in the works of Wassily Kandinsky. Marc Chagall uses many symbols to express his feeling of love. He shows this in flying lovers, and flowers.

The open-spaced sculptures of Henry Moore have an enormous symbolic impact. Look up at Alex Lieberman's massive red structures that dominate the setting, reaching onward, and soaring upward.

Because we are a symbolizing creature, using our conscious part for reality and our unconscious part for infinity, we should become more aware of the creative people who use symbols over and over.

As you go about your daily life, let the symbols you see surround you. Look for them. Can you think of places where you would find symbols?

Language, images, and symbols are the powerful methods used by the brain in action.

Narrative Description of a Brain in Action

A very good way to understand what is happening in people's brains as they go about their daily activities, is to read Virginia Woolf. There's many a reason why Edward

Albee, author of *Who's Afraid of Virginia Woolf*, titled his play that way and has his main character Martha repeat the phrase.

Miss Woolf was a novelist. Her stories are about people and what they are thinking. Experts in human behavior and brain scientists say that she understood the workings of the human mind and expressed it better in literature than anyone else ever has.

The following is a very condensed interpretation, containing none of the magic of the moment or the depth of the narration of *Mrs. Dalloway* by Virginia Woolf. She wrote it showing the interior monologue that goes on and on in every person's brain. This is known as stream of consciousness.

> Mrs. Dalloway takes a walk along the streets of London, to buy some flowers . . . she must do this because Lucy must stay and wait for the men who are coming to take doors off their hinges . . . the walk will be fun . . . she hears a squeaky hinge and recalls a day, she was eighteen, when she opened the door and looked at flowers and thought something dreadful was about to happen . . . she walks and hears Big Ben boom out . . . an hour cannot be replaced . . . why do we love life so much . . . so many desperate people . . . but she loves life . . . especially this month, June . . . thank goodness it is June and the war is over . . . wonder how those who had sons killed are feeling . . . how nice to be out

early in the morning . . . shopkeepers are opening their shops . . . but one must be frugal . . . the party tonight . . . she meets an old friend, Hugh . . . is she wearing an attractive hat? . . . he makes her feel eighteen years old again . . . her husband does not like Hugh . . . or Peter . . . June is showing new leaves . . . she wonders if she should have married Peter . . . she reaches the gates of the Park . . . now she feels young . . . suddenly she feels old . . . she watches the taxis . . . she feels alone . . . she likes to see the taxis and she feels she is nothing . . . but she knows she has an instinct about people . . . can all of this go on without her? . . . the streets of London help her survive because life pulsates here . . . she stops and looks in a glove show window . . . she remembers an uncle who said he always recognized a lady by the shoes and gloves she wore . . . he died . . . she wonders why she has this passion for gloves . . . her daughter does not.

The author goes beneath usual narration to reveal Mrs. Dalloway. Her thoughts show how the mind skips through association, distractions, sounds, sights, environment, and memories. As she continues walking, her thoughts come out of her hopes, fears, emotions, experiences, concerns, and problems.

Your Interior Monologue

The words, images, and symbols that keep tumbling about in your thoughts sometimes need a rest. While you cannot stop your continual interior monologue, you can slow it down with complete relaxation. Feeling uptight? Can't sleep? Restless? Have you been concentrating very hard on a task you are doing? Do personal problems keep whirling around in your brain? Do the following techniques for ten to fifteen minutes. It will refresh your mind, give you a nourishing pause.

1. Think of your brain as a clock ticking away. The ticks become slower and slower. Nothing seems very important. The pendulum slows down. Relax. Take a deep breath. Concentrate on breathing. In and out. Slowly. Relax more. Let thoughts and ideas flow out. Let the clock slow down. Relax. Now rise slowly and go about your business, revitalized.
2. Sit in a comfortable chair, feet flat on the floor, hands still. Start thinking about the top of the head and work your way down to the toes. At each part say, "Relaxed I am—top of head. Forehead. Eyes. Cheeks. Nose. Ears. Mouth. Jaw. Neck. Shoulders. Chest. Arms. Abdomen. Hips. Thighs." Keep saying, "Relaxed I am—knees. Lower legs. Ankles. Feet. Toes." You should now be deeply relaxed.
3. Read this and then close your eyes and do the following. Envision yourself approaching ten stairs leading

down. It is dark. Count the steps backwards. See yourself arriving at the bottom into dazzling, beautiful light. Notice a lovely lake opening before you, stretching to infinity. A small boat is waiting. It looks inviting. You step in and with no energy, float along the calm water to a quiet island. Step out of the boat and walk along a path. Admire the exotic plants, the lush foliage, the beautiful flowers. Walk up a small hill. Sit down on the grass and watch a fountain that sprays delicate jets of water into a marble basin. See a bright white light that surrounds you and fills you with joy and makes you feel happy and calm. Now go back to the boat, float across the water, climb up the stairs.

Thought Control

You are in control of your thoughts. You are the master of your brain. Only one thought at a time can be held. Forget old problems that plague you, such as: What is going to happen to my marriage? My job? Will I graduate? Why do I make so many mistakes? Why am I so tired? If you have a problem, pick a time when you are relaxed and ready to create productive thoughts. If you want to lose ten pounds, get a piece of paper and plan how you are going to do this. If you are worried about external problems, choose a sympathetic friend and talk with him or her. Don't go over unpleasant experiences. The more you think unpleasant thoughts or experiences, the more the message gets deeper and deeper in your brain. It is like playing a tape. The groove becomes stronger in the memory traces. Replace these with new thoughts. Plan new experiences. See yourself in exciting, interesting activities.

The busy, active brain we all have is capable of solving our problems and planning ahead for a productive, successful life.

Read through all the following activities. Do as many as your wish.

Activities

Quickies

1. What two numbers multiplied make 9?
2. Why isn't your nose 12 inches long?
3. What is the similarity between % = @?
4. Describe, out loud, a spiral staircase, without using your hands.
5. Count backwards from 100. Now, in the same manner, recite the alphabet from Z to A. Which was easier for you? Why?
6. Consider the following words. Can you see a picture in your mind?

   Squeeze play
   Zucchini brain
   Cliff hanger
   Raised consciousness

Flower therapy
White paternalism
Black holes
Airport terminal

7. Contemplate. Sit down and quietly watch a sunset, look at a flower, or a painting. Let your mind take over and do what it wants to. Pass no judgment; just let thoughts flow in and out. You are using the right hemisphere of your brain.
8. Sit down at a desk or table. Think of a problem you have, like a deadline to meet. Analyze what action you will take. Write down, in chronological order, how you will get started and resolve the problem. You are using the left hemisphere of your brain.
9. Look at yourself in the mirror. Say, out loud, "I am a complete whole human being. My brain may be divided into parts for special purposes, but it all works in a harmonious way so that I can do anything I want to. I am in control."

Thinkies

1. Read one of William F. Buckley, Jr.'s novels, perhaps *Saving the Queen* or *Stained Glass*. Both are good spy stories with intriguing plots. Buckley is a super-gamesman with words.
2. Try a book by George Simenon. He provides good descriptions of people, and their brains, in action,

showing what they are thinking and what influences their thoughts.

3. The next time you are having a conversation with several people, mentally detach yourself. Try looking into their brains. What is going on in their heads? Can you get clues by watching closely? See the muscles tense as they try to express an idea, then pause while they are getting their ideas straight. Notice eyes that look away while they think as well as the little phrases they use to plot ahead, words like okay.
4. The next time you are engaged in a conversation with one person, turn on your radar. Listen carefully. Lean forward to hear better. Observe. Respond to everything that person is saying, showing complete absorption in his or her conversation. Try to imagine what is going on inside that person's head. What kind of words does he or she use? Is that person seeing pictures or using symbols?
5. Take a walk around your neighborhood. Does anything make you change your detached view of your surroundings? Does the sound of a police siren, children playing ball, or a jogger passing you, take your thoughts away?
6. Take five minutes and try to make a record of your thoughts. Jot them down quickly. Was there anything that influenced them? Did you feel more rational or more dreamy?
7. Listen to music. Do you see anything?

8. Next time you are out on errands, walk through some office buildings and churches. Can you find any symbols?
9. Summarize the main points of this chapter, reviewing to see if you remembered them all.

4

Memory, Mentalists, and Mnemonics

Memory experts at the United Nations put on a spectacular performance. When the organization opened in 1945, visitors were interested in seeing and hearing the delegates, but they were intrigued with the translators. A visitor could put on a receiver and by turning the dial, tune to any of the five official languages being translated by the interpreters.

As the delegates speak, the interpreters simultaneously translate the words so the audience can follow the speech. It cannot be a word for word translation, because some words cannot be translated literally into another language. Phrases must be changed. However, the correct attitude, nuance, and emphasis must be conveyed. Sometimes an interpreter listens for an hour and then gives the complete speech.

Yet, these marvelous memory giants are just as apt to get up from one room, go to another room, look around and wonder what they wanted there. They also mislay the car keys and forget as much as anyone else.

Their key to remembering is motivation. If you want to, you can recall anything. Jerry Lucas, coauthor of *The Memory Book*, wanted to do a dramatic feat for publicity purposes. He memorized hundreds of pages of the Manhattan telephone book and could reel off about 30,000 names along with their telephone numbers.

Training, combined with motivation, is the second key. Memory experts on the stage give remarkable exhibitions. You have probably seen performers circulate among the audience, talk to them, look at their faces, and at sometime during the program, call off all the names of the people in the audience. Harry Lorayne, coauthor of *The Memory Book*, was once on a live television show where he was able to recall the name of every person in the audience. He can remember up to 600 new names at one time. How does he do this?

He has spent years developing his talent, improving and expanding his memory abilities. He is also highly motivated; he makes his living by using his memory. If you went to a party and met thirty new people, could you recall each name and person? What if you were offered $50 a name? How about $100? $500? $1,000?

What would you like to be able to remember? What is

most important to you and would help you in your goals? How many of the following list can you remember?

Faces
Names—social and business
Facts
Telephone numbers
Addresses and zip codes
Appointments
Anniversaries and birthdays
Long digit numbers
Historical dates
Main ideas of every book and article read
Hobbies, habits, and families of associates and friends
Errands without a list
Conversations
Geographical information
Public speaking without notes
Presidents of the United States
States and capitals
A musical composition

With motivation and training, you can do any of the above, and improve on what you have already memorized.

What Is Memory?

A dictionary definition tells us that memory is reproducing or reliving past experiences. Four phases of memory have been recognized: learning, retention, recall, and recognition.

When you learn something new, it leaves an impression on the brain called an engram, or a memory trace. It involves a change in the molecular structure. Electrochemical circuits rearrange themselves to suit the need. Engrams are the pathways to memory.

There are two kinds of memory: short-term and long-term. An example of short-term memory is remembering a telephone number just long enough to dial it. Long-term memory is limitless. It may be with you for life. A short-term memory, stimulated enough and repeated often, will become long-term.

Experiments on aids to memory were done by Dr. Holger Hyden, a neurobiologist at the University of Goteborg, Sweden. He believed that RNA (ribonucleic acid) plays a large role in deciding the amount of protein to be produced in the brain. He tested this theory that RNA in the brain nerve cells makes molecules of protein in order to change the cells to store memory items.

He experimented with rats and mice. First, he taught right-handed rats to become left-handed. When this memory was stored in the rat's brain, the brain was dissected. It was discovered that the amount of RNA had increased. Then he taught mice to perform a task. Afterward they were given medicine which stopped proteins from being produced. On further testing, they had forgotten how to do the newly-taught task.

So, it is possible that protein is an important ally of memory. It is also probable that RNA plays a large role in memory. Experiments have been going on for many years on memory pills that stimulate the brain to produce RNA. In the future, if the tests become conclusive and safe, a memory pill could help you to study for a test or to memorize a speech quickly.

Isaac Asimov, noted writer and scientist, believes that each human brain, in one lifetime, can store 1,000,000, 000,000,000 (one million billion) pieces of information.

How is memory retrieved? No one is quite sure. Some speculation has been given that brain waves, through an electrical activity, scan and search for stored knowledge.

Use your own memory traces to recall a recent experience. Relive a lunch with a friend. Where did you meet? Describe the surroundings. Recall the waiters, the table, the food. How was your friend? How did you feel? In general, you remember what interests you.

Why We Forget—True or False

1. If we keep trying to recall the name of a person and keep thinking about it, we will remember it. False. The

more you worry, the harder it gets. Trying too hard impedes recall. Think about the person. Relax. Usually the memory pops up when you least expect it.

2. Memory worsens with age. This is not necessarily true. Memory skills peak at about twenty years of age, and stay almost unchanged to about age forty-five, when they drop a little. Good recall can continue for a lifetime. It depends more on the individual than on age. If a person is in good health and active, age matters little.
3. You can improve memory by cramming lots of memorization of poems or prose into your brain. False. It may be meaningful to you, but it will not improve your memory. One of the first scientists to investigate this was Dr. William James, psychologist and philosopher in the nineteenth century. Keeping careful track of the time it took him to memorize, he experimented. He learned 158 lines of *Satyr*, by Victor Hugo. Next he memorized, in several weeks, *Paradise Lost*, by Milton. Then he memorized another 158 lines of *Satyr*. The last one took him the longest. Memory is not like a muscle—the more you use a muscle, the stronger it becomes. Memorization exercises do not develop retention; only improving memory skills will do that.
4. During the passage of time, memory dulls. False. What happens *during* that time can cause memory loss. Interference between learning and recall is the culprit. For instance, one student studies his textbook in preparation for an exam the following day and then goes to

sleep. Another student does the same amount of studying but goes to a party that is stimulating and exciting. The first student, without distractions and interference, will usually do better.

5. Good memory means the ability to recall everything. False. It is not important to remember every name, address, and telephone number in your local directory, or last week's shopping list.
6. Constant repetition always improves memory. False. Estimate how many times you have looked at your watch. What does the face look like, the numbers?

Memory Variables

We are each a unique individual. Because of emotion, anger, and individual viewpoint, two people may go through the same experience and remember it very differently.

For example, a man and a woman have a strong and highly emotional argument. These two people may recall two separate and distinct replays of the argument. If they discuss it, it may seem like two different experiences. Each remembers through what he or she saw, and heard, from his or her own point of view.

If the two people then have some pleasant experiences, they may say, "What did we argue about?" Pleasure in each other and happiness may make them forget the disagreeable parts of the argument. Memory traces may change. *We really don't always know if what we remember is accurate.*

Each person remembers an event from his own relative position. Lawrence Durrell shows this brilliantly in *The Alexandria Quartet*, which is a series of four books: *Justine, Balthazar, Mountolive,* and *Clea*. The story takes place in Alexandria, Egypt. Each book covers the same people, place, period of time, and events. But each story is different, depending on the viewpoint of the main character.

Memory may bend to make the past acceptable. Businessmen discuss their large profits on the stock market, not mentioning the losses they have incurred. Do they want to distort the truth? No, they just want to recall the times they proved they were intelligent and made good decisions.

Our memory and ego combine so that we see ourselves as "good" people. We put a rosy glow on the past. We can bend our memory traces to be able to live in the present without the disturbing reminders of past failures.

The Man Who Had the Most Amazing Memory in the World

In his very readable book, *The Mind of a Mnemonist*, A.R. Luria, of the University of Moscow, tells of how he studied an amazing man for nearly forty years.

The man was known only as S. He could remember everything, as long as S wanted to, with perfect comprehension.

How did he do this? S made images and put everything in a visual form. When he went shopping, he could remember dozens of items. He would walk along the streets of Moscow and see each item in his mind. If he was shown many objects, he could immediately recall them all. Long sequences of numbers were presented to him and he would recall all of them with accuracy. When shown a very complicated drawing of a formula, he could draw it at will, and fifteen years later could repeat the drawing to the slightest detail.

He could lower and raise his blood pressure at will. Visualizing himself resting in bed, his pressure would drop. Or, he would imagine himself running to catch a train, and his pressure would go up. If he visualized his right hand on a hot stove, the hand's temperature rose. At the same time he could see his left hand holding ice, thus lowering that extremity's temperature by several degrees.

But to S it became a curse. He often wished he did not have the ability. He would become confused with too many images and found it hard to hold a job.

Although we are not blessed or cursed with the memory abilities of S, we can use many of his skills to advantage.

Ways to Improve and Expand Memory Abilities

Hermann Ebbinghaus, 1850–1909, disagreed with his fellow scientists, who did not believe it was possible to study memory scientifically. He wanted to know the relationship of the time necessary to retain new information to the amount of material to be learned. He made up nonsense words such as dak, dek, col, fup, and ris. After making up sixteen words, he tested recall in various ways.

His conclusion was that recall drops almost immediately. He drew curves showing that if the recall is repeated right away and then again over several days, the recall continues. It is not the number of times repeated, but the time factor that was the most important aid. Repetition is best spread over several days. Initially, try to remember overnight, and then keep repeating what you want to remember for several days.

Winston Churchill would write a speech, take a few days to memorize it, and recite it word for word. His stirring speeches did not sound memorized.

Politicians and leaders are skilled, not only in making speeches, but in remembering names and faces. When Napoleon met a new recruit, he would repeat the name of the soldier and ask a few personal questions. Napoleon knew most of the names of the thousands of soldiers under his command and something special about each one.

A very common reason people cannot remember the name of a new acquaintance is they don't listen or pay attention when the introduction takes place. They did not really forget; there was nothing to recall. If it is noisy and you can't hear, ask the person to repeat his or her name, or even spell it if necessary. Then repeat the name out loud.

Why do we forget where we put our keys or glasses? We

don't pay attention. Say to yourself: "I am now putting my keys in the drawer." "My glasses are on the desk."

Another way to remember is by classification. If people have many items or ideas to recall, they can learn to group together similar ideas and to break down a long list to a few groups.

If a cartographer wanted to be able to remember all the states and their location, he could try to draw a map of the United States from memory. Then he could study a map. Then similar parts could be grouped together.

Cadence, the rhythmic flow of words, is also a good memory jogger. Remember how you learned to spell Mississippi by doing it in a sing-song voice?

One of the msot famous jingles tells us how to remember the days in each month:

Thirty days has September,
April, June and November,
All the rest have thirty-one,
Except February alone,
Which has twenty-eight in line,
Until Leap Year comes for twenty-nine.

Mentalists

Many people have developed into mental giants. They have good memories because it is important to them, and they apply memory skill.

Mentalists have the capacity to see the whole, understand

the parts, see the patterns. Anyone can, with practice.

A highly desirable skill is to read and be able to remember what has been read. Find a book or article you would like to read and be able to recall. Examine the title. What does it tell you? Read any prefaces or introductions; look at any pictures. Read the chapter headings or subtitles. Can you see the purpose of the author? Is there a pattern forming? As you read, stop often and state what the author is saying, in your own words. At the end of the reading, make a statement that summarizes the conclusions reached.

Many fine musicians find it difficult to memorize musical compositions. To do this they begin by taking the music away from the instrument. They study it, analyze for direction, figure out which way the music is moving. They look for notes and phrases that repeat themselves. When they play it, both the brain and the fingers already know it.

Mnemonists

Mnemonists are those who have learned a memory system. The Roman and Greek orators had such a memory system, since speeches were the order of the day.

The speaker would use the memory system of association. He would use his house as the memory aid. For the opening, he would visualize his front door. Then for a second point he would see the foyer. The speech would continue, each idea associated with his house.

Mnemonists today have added many systems. All mnemonic systems are based on visualization. Using "hooks" to visualize a name or a number with an image, is another method. Pictures can be linked together to form a chain, or old memories can be associated with new ideas.

Hook Words

Some words may be remembered because they sound alike. Think of "Dr. Glamb is a lamb." Picture him this way and you will never forget his name.

The more ridiculous the image, the better you will remember it. In remembering people's names, first focus on the person and his or her appearance. Maybe the person has a large nose, ears that stick out, or a beard. Hook the name to a visual picture. Mr. Nelander has a bristly mustache. See his knee (ne) landing (lander) on his mustache.

"How do you do, Gladys Madison." She has a large smile. She looks—glad. She might frown, though, if she is mad at her son. "Hello, Gordon Daniels." See a garden (Gordon) where Dan is yelling (Daniels).

Then reverse the method and make sure that a new acquaintance remembers your name. "My name is Rose Browning. Two colors, that's me." "My name is Pheebe, with two e's together." "I am Adam Washington; my parents hoped I would become President."

Linking

To remember a list of items or objects, link them together by forming visualizations that lead from one item to another.

This forms a memory chain. The best rule to follow is to picture a silly image by exaggerating them.

For example, you have four errands to do. 1. Go to the bank and cash a check. 2. Buy stamps at the post office. 3. Stop by the bakery for a birthday cake. 4. Go to the hardware store for a new garden hose.

First step, going to the bank. See yourself writing out a *check* that is of enormous size. It is so big the teller has to use a huge *stamp* on the back. Now you have linked check to stamps. Picture a mailman with a large *birthday cake* on his head with lighted candles blazing. Now add the link of buying a new garden hose. See the cake and candles and a huge hose dousing water on the candles.

This list can be endless as long as you continue linking each errand or item with individual pictures that are out of context and full of action.

Association

You can remember anything in sequence, if you associate with information you already know. Beginning piano students learn the phrase, "Every good boy does fine." They easily remember the phrase and associate the first letter of each of the five words with the lines of the music staff.

If you want to impress people, tell them what you have learned about memory, listing these key points:

1. Motivation.
2. Training.

3. Pay attention, get it right.
4. Remember what interests you.
5. Spread repetition over several days.
6. Group together similar ideas or items.
7. Rhyme or cadence.
8. See the whole, parts, and patterns.

Visualize a railroad station in order to remember the above.

1. Motivation. You see the train gates closing. You don your Superman outfit and leap over the gate because you are *highly motivated* to get on the train.

2. Training. You see a train painted red, white and blue. It is the wrong *training*.

3. Pay attention. You go back inside the station to the ticket counter. You pay for your ticket with a large check made out to *pay attention*.

4. You remember what interests you. The ticket seller says, "This is an anniversary day for us, so we are paying 10 percent *interest* on ticket prices to all passengers."

5. Spread repetition over several days. You take the money and go to the cafe and watch the cook *spread* peanut butter and jelly over slices of bread, watching him *repeat* his work until you have enough sandwiches to last you *several* days.

6. Group together several items or ideas. You walk around the station, rearranging the furniture, *grouping together* all the chairs in one place.

7. Rhyme or cadence. You hear the announcer call out in a *sing-song* voice, "All aboard for Mis—sis—si—ppi."

8. See the whole, parts, and patterns. Since you are still Superman, you fly over the tracks and see the *whole* train. You fly lower and look into all the sections or *parts*. Then you fly ahead of the train to watch the *pattern* of the tracks.

Numbers

How can you remember numbers more efficiently? Combine association, hook numbers, and pictures, and then link the numbers together.

Numbers are abstract and hard to visualize, so substitution is the name of this game. Associate through words that sound alike or look alike.

For words that sound alike, think of one as gun. It rhymes. Think of five as hive. Try to remember the number 1551. See a large gun (1) shooting into a beehive (5). The bees come out of the hive (5) and grab the gun (1).

Or use words that look like numbers. One looks like a candle, tall and slender. Five could be a foot with five toes. Picture a candle (1) sitting on an enormous foot (5). Wax drops on the foot (5) and kicks the candle (1) high in the air. These systems can also be continued for long digit numbers. Just keep "seeing" the picture for each number, and link each number to the next.

Make up your own hooks and links. They will become part of you and are easy to use. You can use the mnemonic systems to remember whatever you want to—states and capitals, telephone numbers, addresses and zip codes, historical dates, presidents of the United States. The possibilities are infinite.

Activities

Speed reading is a valuable asset. For students who must read many textbooks, for business people with reports to study and remember, for doctors, lawyers, engineers who must keep up in their field through technical papers, this is a practical and useful tool.

The purpose of speed reading is to read faster, with more accuracy and greater comprehension.

The basic techniques are:

1. Preview
2. Practice
3. Concentration
4. Review.

Before reading, skip through the material, looking for main points. Try to catch the thoughts while forcing yourself to read faster. Guess at words you don't know and look them up later; establish a pace.

Do not move your head as you read to yourself; make no lip movements. Don't use a pencil or a finger as a pointer. Go back over the material only when you have completed the reading. Begin by reading magazines and newspapers, which contain easy-to-understand material.

Eyes do not naturally follow the reading line steadily;

they stop, read, stop again, then zig-zag along. At the end of the line, the eyes must sweep back to the beginning of the following line, from right to left. Speed reading teaches how to reduce these stops and sweeps.

Our eyes have peripheral vision, which means we have the ability to see the right and left sides of our view even while looking straight ahead. Look out a window but keep your head straight, without turning. See how much you can see on each side.

When you are speed reading, you will use this ability. Try to read looking down the middle of the material. You can practice by drawing a faint center line down a newspaper article from top to bottom. As you read, try not to let your eyes deviate very much from this line. Don't stare in a fixed gaze; relax your eyes and go down the column. With practice you will be able to read more and more of the left and right sides of the line without moving the eyes.

Adjust to the difficulty of the material and don't worry about comprehension at this time; it will come. Just keep reading, and at the end review what you were reading—subject, main points, and conclusion.

This same method can be used for everything from taking exams to filling out employee forms when applying for a job. Speed read the complete text, by skimming down the pages quickly. First see it as a whole. Then see the parts and complete the answers. Usually your first answer is correct. Skip over what you don't know and return to unanswered questions if there is time.

Speed reading techniques must be continually practiced in order to enable the reader to "go faster." You can easily learn to read at twice your present rate while doubling comprehension, efficiency, and recall.

5

Head in the Right Direction

I look at the earth, the hills and the seas,
the moon, the sun, and stars in the sky,
I feel the touch of a cool, soft breeze.
I look in the mirror and wonder—who am I?

The image in the mirror shows the external person. The mirror reflects a body and face that others recognize as an individual, and identify by name as a certain person.

What goes on inside is not so easily revealed. That which gives each person a unique personality, particular behavior patterns, and especially hopes and dreams cannot be so easily seen.

Parents, relatives, friends, neighbors, teachers—all of them influence the development of the child. This conditioning goes on constantly. While the many theories on differences between males and females vary, Dr. Estelle Ramey, an endocrinologist at Georgetown University of Medicine, thinks that although sex hormones determine whether a person will be a boy or girl, after birth the brain takes over and overrides the hormone system. She feels it is not the sex of the child that makes a boy more aggressive or goal seeking than his sister: It is the conditioning of males in the family and in society that is responsible for role playing.

Ivan Pavlov, in his famous experiments, showed how conditioning works. He would ring a bell when giving food to a dog. This was repeated many times. The dog then learned to salivate at the sound of the bell whether or not food was present. He had been conditioned. In much the same way we are all conditioned to answer the telephone or a doorbell. And we are conditioned to many other things as well.

What you have been conditioned to believe can help to cure many health problems. Dr. H.K. Beecher of Harvard, did some placebo (sugar pills with no medicinal value) experiments that have since become well known. He was interested in placebo effectiveness against pain. When certain patients were given the sugar pills and told they would help, thirty-three persons out of every one hundred patients found relief.

Scientists at the University of California, San Francisco,

have wondered why placebos work. Dr. Howard L. Fields and his associates thought it might be that placebos trigger the release of the chemical endorphin, and activate the body's natural pain killer. Tested on dental patients who had just had an extraction, about one-third had less pain after being injected with a placebo.

In the December 1980 issue of *Psychology Today* an interesting experiment done by two assistant professors of the State University of New York at Albany. George Smelch and Richard Felsen appeared. The professors wanted to know if students believe their superstitions have an actual power, or whether they helped them psychologically by relieving stress in certain circumstances.

Questionnaires were given to 270 sociology students in Albany, New York, and 180 students at University College, Dublin, Ireland. Among the questions were do you do anything special for luck when you take exams? Engage in sports contests? Prepare for an important meeting, interview, or date? Does anything you do make you believe you can succeed?

Out of the 450 students, 70 percent used something that he or she believed gave them a better chance. They carried good-luck charms, crossed fingers, had a lucky number, knocked on wood, wore special attire, had special jewelry or coins. Forty-three percent thought they had a lucky number that helped them win in card playing. One football player had to be the last one out of the locker room and on to the playing field because it had been lucky for him before. Superstition or conditioning to magic beliefs may be below the threshold of awareness. That is why the student is doing it; it is deeply ingrained in him to play it safe. Not sure if the "magic" works or not, he is willing to try to relieve stress and win.

Your Self-Image

Self-image is your concept of yourself. It is a picture that we carry in our subconscious, and while we are not always aware of it, it determines what we can and cannot do. It sets limits, so that we are always behaving in accordance with it. If a young man has decided he is unpopular, shy, or not a good student, he will do everything possible to maintain that self-image.

The self-image develops from a total build-up of the past. Every experience and person in our life is painted on our personal canvas. Once we get "our image," it stays with us. Everything we do is consistent and harmonious with our self-image. It guides us in all our behavior.

Prescott Lecky was an early researcher in the field of the self-image. He became a member of the faculty of Columbia University, New York, in 1924. Because he was an educator, he was able to test his theories on many students. After years in active research, Lecky was convinced that poor learning abilities were due to a student's self-conception.

He believed that all people have an idea system, that is the ideas a person has about himself must be consistent with the concept others have of him. Otherwise, the ideas are rejected. Lecky listened to students and their statements, such as, "I am a poor speller," "Mathematics is not anything I can ever understand," and "Foreign languages are not for me." He thought that students who expressed these ideas about themselves did not lack ability; they did lack a good self-image.

Being fat today is a major concern of many people. How many overweight people heard, when they were growing up, such statements as: Clean your plate. Remember the starving children in other lands. Everyone in our family is fat. You're tired and had a busy day, sit down and eat a nice piece of chocolate cake. Guilt, discipline, and rewards were all programmed into the self-image.

Many of these "fat" images were created in very early years. Up to the age of three children accept everything told to them by their parents. This can continue to the age of six. Children have no freedom of choice, and less critical judgment.

Even when the children are older, the self-image continues to imprint what they have been told onto their brains: "Your room is a mess and you will always be a sloppy person," "Your poor grades in school show you are stupid," "Why don't you shape up and be more like your father?"

What we all need to do is to develop an acceptable self-image that works. It must be one which provides self-esteem and the ability to express ourselves freely, without worrying about what other people expect from us or if they are judging us. We need a self-image that makes us feel good and gives us self-confidence.

Changing your self-esteem does not mean becoming a perfect person; it simply means improving your own image. To do this, think of yourself more honestly. Free yourself of past failures and the negative programming fed to you as a child, and you will become more vital and alive and will achieve new goals that will be of value and satisfying.

When you change your self-image you change both behavior and personality. By expanding your potential, you open up a whole new range of opportunities and possibilities.

How to Change Your Self-Image

Forget past bad memories and remember good experiences. When something doesn't work out and you feel put down and think of yourself as a failure, recall the many times you *did* succeed in an accomplishment and felt good about it. Start accepting yourself as you are. You are a human being, who has needs and desires. Remember, no one is perfect or imperfect. Everyone has strengths and weaknesses. Build on your strengths. You already have certain abilities, and while you can't create new ones, you can improve your skills and expand and release the abilities that you have. You are the only one responsible for your life. Assume control and get your head in the right direction.

EIGHT STEPS TO CHANGE YOUR SELF-IMAGE

1. Understand yourself.
2. Set goals.
3. Do not pass judgment on yourself.
4. See yourself in winning situations.
5. Don't be held back by fear of making mistakes.
6. Use positive words of affirmation.
7. Relax.
8. Trust your brain.

1. Understand Yourself.

After you finish reading this chapter, write a paragraph describing yourself. Don't describe your physical appearance; detail what you are like as a person. Do you feel you can be yourself at all times? Can you just relax and be "you" when you are with other people? Do you wear a mask at the job, presenting a different face to fellow employees?

Write down any programming you may have received as a child that you carry around today. It need not be negative. Perhaps you received a lot of love and security. Just try to write down accurately how you feel about yourself. First hunches are usually best. You will see your self-image appearing in your words.

You might start by such thoughts as: I see myself as the kind of person who . . . My parents always seemed to treat me as . . . At school I found my teachers and friends . . . When I think about myself deeply, I see. . . .

Now start looking at yourself as a new person. Believe in the process of change. We are always developing, becoming, and growing.

2. Set Goals.

During World War II, Dr. Norbert Wiener, Professor of Mathematics at M.I.T., started studying and doing research on the relationship of man to machines. He called this subject cybernetics, from the Greek word *kybernetes*, meaning "steersman."

Wiener had been working on developing goal seeking mechanisms. For instance, a machine, such as a missile or electronic computer would have a goal and keep on working, correcting itself if necessary, until the target had been reached, and the mission accomplished.

Then Wiener translated this into the field of human behavior. He believes that humans are goal-seeking and goal-striving with built-in mechanisms to make corrections or adjustments. It works automatically; it just has to be set.

Many years ago, Mark G. Harris set a goal for himself. He had been sick and was told to retire and rest. He became bored and tired of hearing his cronies talk about life being over at retirement and how older people could no longer do many of the things they used to do. Harris took this as a personal challenge. He was sixty-five years old and had never played golf in his life. He decided to take up the game and become an expert at it. His goal was established. At the end of four years he was shooting in the seventies. Then he set a new goal: to develop a new system of putting. He practiced, correcting and adjusting as he worked, and then put on remarkable demonstrations. Sports writers started calling him the world's best on the putting green. Then he wrote a best-seller, *New Angles On Putting*, which is still read and followed by many golfers.

What are your goals? At the end of this chapter, write them down. Do not, at this moment, be concerned with how you will accomplish them; just think of what you want to do, not what others have said you should do. Think of the following: habits you would like to change, sports in which you would like to improve; things you would like to accomplish, such as finding a mate, selling a book, earning straight A's in a course you are taking; fears you wish to be rid of, such as fear of flying, heights, or darkness. Your goals may be more philosophical, such as asserting yourself more frequently, having more energy, or looking forward to each day with zest and enthusiasm.

3. Do Not Pass Judgment on Yourself.

Never pass judgment on yourself. It programs you the wrong way, and has negative effects. Forget statements such as: "Why did I make that stupid mistake yesterday?" "Why can't I get more done?" "What's the matter with me?"

Let's say a young man is playing tennis. His first serve is too long. The second is too wide. He might start saying to himself, "What a terrible serve I have. Why can't I get it in the court?'' He might continue negative thoughts when he doesn't get the hit he wants. He may think, ''I didn't turn my wrist over correctly. I didn't follow through or watch the ball.'' As this continues the tennis player keeps judging himself and his muscles tighten. Finally the player starts thinking: I am a terrible tennis player. I don't do anything well. What a stupid person I am.

Do not pass judgment on yourself. W. Timothy Gallwey explains this in his excellent book, *The Inner Game of Tennis*. He says that *you become the person you think you are*. He suggests we really know how to make a good lob, serve, and return; it is inborn in us. And so he gives valuable suggestions on quieting the mind and concentrating. His insights into how to be aware of the inner game of tennis—or what goes on in the head—can be applied to any sport and any situation in life.

Program yourself for using your natural abilities. Program a good self-image. See yourself in winning situations, and you will win.

4. See Yourself in Winning Situations.
Create new images of yourself in your memory storage areas. See yourself in winning situations. Ask a new friend for a date and receive an enthusiastic response and a big smile. Ask the boss for a promotion and get it.

When football player Robert ''Rocky'' Bleier talks to youth groups, he likes to sum up his philosophy by saying that the one who thinks he can win, sooner or later, will.

He had many reasons for not being a winning football star. As a youth in Appleton, Wisconsin, he had Osgood-Schlatter's disease. His bones were growing faster that his muscles. He was told he could not play sports for three years. This did not stop him; he was out to win. The second year of his disease, he joined the seventh grade basketball team and in high school earned eleven letters in three sports and a football scholarship to Notre Dame. His season with the Pittsburgh Steelers, on graduation, was short because he was soon drafted and sent to Vietnam, where a grenade shattered the bones of his right foot. Many operations were necessary. The doctors said he would never play football again; he would be lucky to walk without a limp.

Rocky was sent to the Irwin Army Hospital, Fort Riley, Kansas. On his own, he went back into training. Every morning he would walk or run several agonizing miles and in the evenings he would sprint and lift weights. In July, 1970, he appeared at the Steelers' Training Camp. He played in only one game the first year. By 1974 he went to the Super Bowl and made a winning play. He went on to more spectacular wins, but one of his greatest pleasures is working with handicapped children and teaching them that being strong and fast is not always the answer; a person who wins is often the one who believes he can.

On his eightieth birthday, Aaron Copland showed no signs of giving up reaching his goals. He has never lost his dream, vision, and desire to win success as a conductor.

Born in 1900 in Brooklyn, his parents were hard-working Jewish emigrees from Russia who lived over the store they owned. While one sister played the piano and an older brother the violin, the family did not take music seriously, and they could not understand Aaron's need for music.

But Copland took his musical career seriously and was enthusiastic. He could see himself as a world-famous composer. He started taking piano lessons at age thirteen. He eventually wrote books, gathered musicians together to play and hear the new music, lectured, taught at Berkshire Music Center, Tanglewood, and achieved his vision as a successful conductor. He always saw himself as a musician. Aaron Copland is a winner; he has always seen himself as one.

First to admit he owes his success to concentration and visualization, Jack Nicklaus is a winner. He knows what to do to win and does it. He closes off the outside world. Then he sees, in his head, pictures of his winning shot. He never hits a golf ball without doing this. He sees the ball where he wants it to be. Next he visualizes how the ball will get there, the path it will take, how it will roll on landing. He knows how to win and sees himself as a winner. He has proven it over and over again.

Runners keep looking for ways to improve, to better their mileage, their time, to win against themselves. Dr. John "Pat" O'Shea, a world famous exercise physiologist, says the way to improve is to expect your performance to get better. Your brain controls what you achieve, whether it is success or failure.

He claims "self-image" is the key. We either see ourselves as losers or winners. He believes that positive thoughts must be dynamic. O'Shea recommends repeating affirmative statements over and over daily, or writing them on three-by-five cards, putting them in your line of vision, and reading them aloud several times a day. An affirmation should start with "I am," not "I will." It should be in the present tense. Hold it in your memory; what we keep in our mind we tend to become.

5. Don't Be Held Back by Fear of Making Mistakes. Artist Robert Motherwill would often paint hundreds of pictures before he finished one that suited him. It wasn't that he thought he was making hundreds of mistakes; he was trying to get a certain idea on canvas. He had a specific goal and high standards of perfection.

The great scientist, Thomas Alva Edison, did thousands of experiments along the way to inventing the electric light bulb. They were not failures; they were necessary steps to arrive at his goal.

Fear and feelings of failure are not part of fate; they come from within the brain and show a lack of confidence.

Instead of thinking of mistakes and failures, remember that when you are achieving a goal there will be corrections and adjustments along the way.

6. Use Positive Words of Affirmation.

Forget the past and any negative programming. From now on believe in yourself. Make positive statements of affirmation to yourself about your self-image.

Words of affirmation can be used in several ways. Try looking in the mirror and saying them to yourself. Write them down. Say them out loud. Put them on tape and play them back.

Each statement of affirmation should contain one thought. Try some of the following:

I have confidence in myself.
I like myself; I'm great.
I have the ability to do whatever I want to do.
Everything I (insert your name) do is a success.
I (your name) am capable of handling anything that comes my way.
I (your name) am in control of my thoughts.
I have infinite potential.

Think of your own words of power and affirmation, whatever helps you feel good about yourself.

The French pharmacist, Émile Coué, experimented in the 1920s with the power of suggestion in order to reach the inner power of the mind. He came up with the following famous saying one should repeat every day. "Every day, in every way, I'm getting better and better."

It works.

7. Relax.

Brain waves are the activity level of your brain. The pattern varies depending on what you are thinking, if you are asleep or if you are meditating.

Beta. Here is the most active brain wave pattern, with thirteen or more vibrations per second. At the beta level you are aware and awake, responding to stimuli around you. You are thinking rationally. This is the action level of the brain.

Alpha. These waves have from seven to thirteen vibrations per second. Here is the part of your brain level you can only reach through relaxation. In this level you use your creativity; your inspirations may occur; your dreams of the future take place; you experience feelings of peace and tranquility.

Theta. These waves have four to seven cycles per second. Only masters of meditation reach this deep level of relaxation.

Delta. With one to four cycles per second, this is the state of unconsciousness or deep sleep.

Through relaxation and meditation you reach your subconscious during the alpha level of brain activity. Since your self-image is in the subconscious, this is the only way to reach it.

Try the following relaxation exercise. Sit comfortably in a chair, feet flat on the floor, hands relaxed in your lap. Breathe deeply several times. Relax your body from head to toe. Let all the tension ooze out. Keep breathing deeply. Close your eyes.

Now create your special place where you will feel at ease. It can be anywhere. Think of a cabin in the woods, floating on a cloud, or going down the Nile River on a barge. In your special place you will have everything you need to achieve your goals.

Picture a big overstuffed chair. Try it for comfort. Feel yourself settling into it. Now create your surroundings, furnishing them to your special taste. Perhaps they will contain all books ever published and a large television screen that will show anything you want to see. Anyone you want to talk to can appear.

Be sure to visualize a garbage disposal where you can throw away all fears and anxieties.

There may be some items in your special place that you didn't plan. There will be a need for them. Your special place may change. Let it happen.

Look around, see and feel the surroundings. You can come here anytime and plan for the future. Believe in your goals and work them out in your special place. Don't try too hard; let it happen. Don't force thoughts, let them come to you. You are now at the alpha awareness level. You are reaching your subconscious and thus your self-image.

Do this for about fifteen minutes at a time. When you are finished, open your eyes, stretch, and relax for a few minutes.

When you are relaxed, and your muscles are not tense, you cannot feel hostile, hurt, angry, or afraid. Tensing muscles put us in action to respond to persons and events. If no tension results, and no muscles become tight, there are no destructive feelings. Relaxation is a natural tranquilizer.

Many relaxation techniques and treatments are used at UCLA's Pain Clinic. Dr. David Bressler Dr. C. Norman Shealy have worked with many of them, and they think you may have more control over the function of your body than you think possible. Perhaps your body can do anything you want. Right now your body may be responding to whatever you have told it, in ways you may not have consciously directed it—good health or illness, for example.

HOLISTIC HEALTH

A growing number of doctors and health professionals are working in the field of holistic health, where the prevention of sickness is stressed. There are no twenty-minute fast in-and-out appointments. The doctor wants to know the patient because the onset of an illness is not always isolated; it can relate to stress, life-style changes, emotional upsets, and traumatic experiences. Confidence and trust between doctor and patient is imperative, because holistic health treats the entire person, emphasizing a good attitude, assuming responsibility for your own health, and encouraging a positive and a tranquil state of mind.

When illness occurs, the doctor will help the patient use his body to heal itself doing techniques that help the body's natural immune system to function. The patient takes an active role in getting well because holistic doctors and health professionals believe the body has an innate power to heal.

Holistic health is more than a slight change in medical practice. It encompasses a whole new concept and viewpoint. It is controversial and not accepted by all health professionals, partly because many medical people have not studied it. Medical changes come slowly, cautiously and with skepticism, as has often been the case in new medical or health findings.

THE MIND CAN DO ANYTHING

Dr. Irving Oyle, doctor, author, and instructor at the University of California, Santa Cruz, participated at a seminar, *The Mind Can Do Anything*, in Honolulu, Hawaii, June, 1979. Also involved in the two day seminar were R. Buckminster Fuller, designer and geometrician; Uri Geller who moves objects without touching them; Thelma Ross, Ph.D., medical psychologist; and Olga Worrell, Ph.D., a spiritual healer.

Oyle, who practices holistic health, has some innovative ideas about what your brain can do. He wants to discover the outer limits of how the brain can influence healing. He believes that you can think yourself sick, and you can think yourself well. Change your thinking and you change the state of your body.

The body has great power to heal itself because it is a

self-repairing mechanism. Inner belief is the largest factor in healing power. This comes about by activating your immune system. He claims there are four different immunization processes ready and working to attack and destroy cancer. The stronger the belief, the sooner the patient gets well. He discussed four weapons against cancer: (1) surgery, (2) radiation, (3) chemotherapy, and (4) fighting back using the immune system.

How do you heal the body in holistic health? There are two main ways: meditation and visualization.

Dr. Oyle spoke of Dr. Carl Simonton, Director of the Cancer Counseling and Research Center in Fort Worth, Texas, who has used these treatments with success. Simonton became frustrated as a radiologist working with terminal cancer patients. He developed his theories at the Oncology Departments at the University of Oregon Medical School and Travis Air Force Base.

Again, these treatments are highly controversial and not accepted by everyone. Still not proven, more attention is being paid because the methods are saving lives. Dr. Simonton emphasizes that his treatments are not to play down the important role of the doctor and health professionals, but instead work with them in new medical treatments. He does not want patients to use only his psychological treatments and ignore traditional methods such as chemotherapy, surgery, and radiation. Patients should not overlook the accumulated data of the medical community.

His techniques utilize the brain beginning wth meditation and working toward mental imagery or visualization.

First, meditation. Very relaxing and therapeutic, the body enters a state of ease without stress. You gain control of your conscious mind. At first, thoughts dart here and there, and it is hard to settle down. Try to be aware of your breathing, concentrating on it and stopping the brain's thoughts from flying around. Give full attention to what you are doing, it improves concentration. The following is the meditation exercise steps used by Dr. Simonton:

1. Try to meditate three times daily for ten to fifteen minutes.
2. Find a quiet room where you can be alone, feet flat on the floor, and close your eyes.
3. Be aware of your breathing and as you exhale say, "relax."
4. Start at your head and work your way down the body, feeling relaxation as you progress. Tense muscles if necessary and then make them relax.
5. When you feel your body is completely relaxed, rest for a few minutes.
6. Then open your eyes and continue your normal activities, if you are just trying to relax. If you are trying to heal your body, now is the time to practice visual imagery.

How does one use visual imagery to heal? For the terminal cancer patient, during the meditation he pictures his own cancer and destroys it through his immune system. If he is undergoing chemotherapy, he should try to see the drug coming into his body, poisoning the cancer cells, and cleaning them out of his body. If he is receiving radiation, he should visualize bullets hitting and destroying the cancer cells.

A patient with a cancerous tumor should see it shrinking, and the body getting healthy. Visualize the cancer getting smaller, the dead cells leaving the body, flushed out through the the kidneys and liver and eliminated further through the urine and bowel. See the cancer all gone.

Visualize the white blood cells, defenders of the body, going to the cancer and destroying it. One patient said he saw his white cells as white knights, and during meditation would line them up and have them charge, killing the cancer cells with their lances. Another patient thought of the white cells as fish, swimming around and eating the cancer cells. Another saw the white cells as sharks, voraciously eating cancers.

Dr. Simonton tells his patients to think of white cells as strong and aggressive and cancer cells as weak and confused. A patient can talk to the white cells, asking them to help him and to flow through his body.

Do these treatments work?

Dr. Simonton had success with his first patient while he was at the USAF Medical Center. The patient was sixty-one years old and had throat cancer. He could not eat and could hardly swallow saliva. A treatment employing meditation and visual imagery was started. The patient who was considered terminal and not expected to live long, one and a half years later was alive and had no sign of cancer.

Remembering that Dr. Simonton is working with terminal cancer patients, anyone he saves is a success story. Many have lived. In 1973, using X-ray and visual imagery, 128 cases were successfully cured. Cancer patients come from all over the world to the Cancer Counseling and Research Center in Fort Worth, Texas. They have been told they are incurable; most traditional medical help has been done, or it is too late. In trying his treatments, 159 patients were still alive after four years. Of the patients who died, many lived longer than those receiving the usual treatments for terminal patients.

These techniques can be used for ulcers, irregular heartbeat, high blood pressure, arthritis, and perhaps many more health problems. The field is still in the experimantal stages.

For those wishing to know more information about this, read *Getting Well Again* by Dr. O. Carl Simonton, M.D., Stephanie Mathews-Simonton, and James Creighton.

8. Trust Your Brain.

You do have an amazing brain. Billions of cells are within to help you correlate information, remember and recall, make decisions, solve problems, improve your health, and relax your body. Only with your brain can you change your self-image, accomplish goals, and do whatever you want to do.

Activities

1. Did you speed read the last chapter? If so, how do you feel about speed reading?
2. List your six best talents:
   1.
   2.
   3.
   4.
   5.
   6.
3. Try to answer the question asked at the end of the following story.

   Riding a train one day through Massachusetts, Oliver Wendell Holmes could not find his ticket. He looked through all his pockets, sure that he had bought one. The conductor said, "Hey, Mr. Holmes, that's okay. I know you. Don't worry about finding your ticket. Someone will turn it in." Mr. Holmes said in some dismay, "That is not my problem. Where am I going?"

   Where are you going?

6

The Expanding Brain

To a great extent you have little control over many of the stimuli that reach you during your daily activities. The television program your family insists on watching, the personalities you encounter in working, the ideas a classroom teacher expounds are forced on you. But in a broad sense, you can decide which ideas, sights and sounds, and persons will stimulate you and cause you to think, react, and respond.

You do choose what books you will read, the friends with whom you associate, the people you discuss ideas with, the music you hear, the entertainment you prefer, the newspapers and journals you study, the places you go, and the events you participate in. Since you are what you think, remember, see, and hear, and since you can choose what stimuli will arouse your mind to think, you do have a great amount of control over what will stimulate and motivate you.

All experiences and actions, all thoughts and stimuli change and alter us to some extent. Each day we become a slightly different person, depending on what has happened to us.

When you choose a variety of stimuli, you expand your senses, and you thus expand your mind.

Let's say you attend a local community program on Mexico. In one evening you might see exhibits of handcrafts and the colorful art of Mexicans, hear a mariachi band, watch waiters and entertainers dressed in gay costumes, see a Mexican film, and enjoy tacos and enchiladas. You would have a pleasant and effective evening learning about Mexico.

Or, you are studying history and want to know more about Hitler. Books help, and newspapers and pictures from that time make the news real. But a tape of Hitler's voice provides an additional powerful description of the man.

Surround yourself with books, magazines, pamphlets, pictures, charts, maps, globes, kits, records, tapes, clippings, slides, films, filmstrips, models, and sculpture. The more materials used, the greater the senses are stimulated, and a more complete and enjoyable learning experience occurs.

When you touch, look, listen, taste, and smell you identify and associate in an expanded way. When you increase your sensory input, you expand your thinking.

Everytime you do any of the following you grow, change, and increase your creative potential:

analyze — communicate — compare — create — design — develop — discover — discuss — evaluate — explore — interpret — invent — judge — listen — plan — process — read — test — translate — watch — write.

Can you add more to the above list?

Knowledge is transmitted every time we do any of these functions. Interest leads to information and then to inspiration. Become a lifetime learner, one who is open to new people, experiences, and ideas.

One out of five persons in the United States is involved in a training or educational course. It has been estimated that scientists, engineers, and business professionals may have to reeducate themselves at least three times during their working years. Much of the knowledge in their fields becomes obsolete every ten years.

The lifetime learner who wishes to keep up on varied interests is aware of stimulating activities in the community. This individual visits museums, art galleries, libraries; he or she joins community organizations and watches good television. In addition, he or she attends local groups that meet for specialized reasons, such as politics, neighborhood boards, or community improvement. Many people today are not only taking adult education courses and attending seminars and conferences, but are enthusiastic about special courses on cooking exotic foods, writing poetry, listening to opera, and studying literature. They continue to expand their minds and by doing so, renew themselves.

Self-Renewal

John W. Gardner, in his remarkable book, *Self-Renewal*, uses the title as an expression of the inquiring mind. Mr. Gardner gives a new insight into how to live, looking forward to vitality and maturity. Renewal, as he describes it, is change with purpose that is interwoven with values and becomes a framework of innovation that grows and flourishes with freshness. The person involved in self-renewal must have not only the courage to try but also the courage to fail.

A person who keeps renewing has the freedom to choose as well as the freedom to make decisions, disagree, and be flexible.

How people are motivated, and what their commitments and values are gives meaning to their lives. Human beings are complex; each has his own needs and follows them, but at times everyone can be utterly selfless. When a person relates to something larger than himself, he finds more values along with a more meaningful life. One of any person's greatest needs is to relate to something beyond himself.

Life for the renewing person is not one of pleasure seeking and self-gratification. It makes use of one's powers and abilities to reach out for independence of thought, freedom of action, the capacity to learn, to aspire, and to love.

Peak Experiences

One of the outstanding spokesmen for humanistic psychology and optimism in achieving the highest levels of human awareness was Abraham H. Maslow. He was professor of psychology at Brooklyn College, Chairman of the Department of Psychology at Brandeis University, and President of the American Psychological Association from 1967 to 1968.

Much of his work was based on a holistic psychological approach. Man must be studied as a whole; everything in a person is related to everything else, and the entity is more than any of its parts.

In his studies of many people, he looked for those who were living fully, able to concentrate effectively, to be completely absorbed in what they were doing. He called them self-actualizers. They are objective in observation, able to judge people with accuracy, listen well, they find work a pleasure and a necessity because commitment is a requirement to them. Self-actualizers are at peace with themselves, feel they are in control of their lives and actions, and self-discipline comes easily to them.

When self-actualizers were interviewed, they spoke of

having special experiences, of times when they felt exhilarated and in tip-top condition. Maslow, on further investigation, found that most people have these peak experiences. In fact, he had trouble finding anyone who did not have peak experiences. This can happen through a sports achievement, a fine sexual experience—anything that seems perfect at the moment.

Don't just sit there and wait for a peak experience. It doesn't happen that way. It is spontaneous and does happen to everyone. We don't know how to hold on to it, so we often forget it. There is no way to create it. It comes out of serenity, as a source and moment of greatness, when a person feels completely integrated, alert, and creative.

Acquiring lifetime learning habits, maintaining an inquiring mind, using the techniques of self-renewal, and having peak experiences are all excellent ways to expand the brain into new channels of discovery and increase the quality of living.

The New Brain

Has the brain stopped evolving and reached its potential? No scientist, no brain researcher, no expert in human development has said that the brain has achieved its potential. Instead, there is a growing awareness that the possibilities of brain growth are infinite.

The man who has contributed the most in this field is

Tielhard de Chardin, theologian, scientist, paleontologist, and author. Born in 1881, he entered the Jesuit order at eighteen. Some of the ideas he expressed later in life seemed unorthodox to the church, and he was eventually forbidden to teach or write on philosophical subjects. His manuscripts were left with a friend and published after Chardin's death.

Chardin believed that the universe is consistent and very logical, and that it is still growing and changing. For billions of years the universe has been continuing to evolve, and Chardin saw this as the way things will continue. He believed that evolution has a direction toward growth, improvement, awareness of consciousness, complexity, modifications, and especially change. The brain, being part of the universe, is constantly perfecting itself.

The Brain and "Super-Learning"

Sheila Ostrander and Lynn Schroeder, with Nancy Ostrander have written the thought-provoking book *Super-Learning*. The book discusses how to use our potentials better, with less stress. But it is much more than that. Several new systems on learning have been put together, all presenting a holistic viewpoint, seeing the person as an entity, not just someone who wants to speak German, play better golf, or make better business decisions. The ideas for the new system came from doctors in Bulgaria, Spain, and Germany, and the originator is Dr. Georgi Lozanov, Bulgarian doctor and psychiatrist. He, like so many, believes the brain has unlimited potential for learning and memory. He says his ideas came from physiology, hypnosis, autogenics, music, sleep learning, and much more. The system is called the Bulgarian Rapid-Learning Method.

Fifteen professionals, from age twenty-two to sixty, came to Sofia, Bulgaria, in the mid 1960s. They stayed at the Institute of Suggestology all day and into the evening. According to Dr. Lozanov, the theory of Suggestology supposes that states of consciousness for developing learning, of intuitive behavior, and of healing can be altered. These people had come somewhat reluctantly to learn French. The leader read French phrases with different tones of voice. Classical music could be heard in the background. The participants sat quietly, with eyes closed, listening to the teacher wheedle, cajole, and change from a soft voice to a harsh and demanding tone. Then the participants took a test that surprised them. On an average, they learned 1,000 new French words in one day. Usually people learn 50 to 150 new words in an intense learning situation or from 50 to 150 new pieces of information in one day.

In the USSR, it was said that 1,000 people learned a new language in twenty-four days, and a history course in a few months. Speed learning increases learning speed from five to fifty times. Hardly any effort is required by the student, and no elaborate equipment is needed.

In 1976 seventeen public schools in Bulgaria were using the system. High school algebra was done by third graders.

The pupils could do two school years in four months. Everyone liked it, thought it was fun, and it made them feel good. There were no failures, no poor students. Dr. Cecilia Pollack of Lehmann College, New York, observed school number 122 in Sofia. She watched nine-year-old students solving abstruse algebra problems, and first graders reading well beyond their level and discussing folk tales normally used in a third grade.

The Bulgarian Rapid-Learning Method has been tried in the United States. Americans have analyzed the system to determine how it works. Some of the findings included pacing of the material to the music, expanding a person's perception of time, self-image therapy, altered states of consciousness, rhythmical breathing, the freedom of stress, and the feeling of pleasure.

The authors state that the two real reasons for the success are: (1) the relaxed state of being, because meditation is used; and (2) the synchronized rhythm, since certain music brings a relaxed state. Information, voice tones, breathing, music are all in harmony. Learning takes place.

The Amazing Brain

You do have an amazing brain. Sir John Eccles, 1963 Nobel Prize Winner in physiology and medicine for his discoveries about the nervous system, did his research in neurophysiology. It is basic to comprehending how neurons interact with each other which led to a better understanding of the higher functions of the brain. Eccles predicted that in the next century most scientists will be researching the brain to prevent mental retardation and mental disorders, to improve abilities of memory and learning, to cure violent and aggressive behavior, to help the body heal itself through the brain's direction, and to avoid stress and tension. The fields of hypnosis, parapsychology, and human potential will be more fully explored.

Neurological scientists at UCLA are researching the possibility of the brain having limitless potential. Researchers are trying to develop methods to better enable use of the senses to smell, see, listen, and experience the environment more fully through more kinesthetic and tactile abilities. Kinesthetic abilities could improve the sensation of movement in the muscles, tendons, and joints. Tactile improvement would make a person more perceptive to touch. Increased sensual abilities would help you be more aware of the environment, to be more sensitive to what is happening around you, and increase awareness of yourself.

Exploring and activating the enormous power of your brain is the most exciting game in the world. The more you ask of your brain, the more it can do, the easier it will do it, and the quicker it will respond.

You are your brain. Your brain is you. Here is the very center of your existence. Keep playing the brain game all of your life.

Activity

Dr. Art Ulene, who frequently appears on television, and Dr. David Bressler of the UCLA Medical School Pain Center suggest having animals act as guides for us. Drs. Irving Oyle and Carl Simonton also recommend this exercise. It is fun and relaxing. It is a way of talking to your inner self and often receiving excellent advice.

1. Sit, feet flat on the floor. Close your eyes and be comfortable.
2. Think of a place you like, where you can relax.
3. Find a friend, animal, person, plant, bird, or presence. Watch for it, look around until you find it.
4. Make friends with it. Talk to it. Get acquainted. Feed it.
5. Ask if it will answer your questions.
6. They answer in simple ways, so listen carefully.
7. It must believe in you or it won't take you seriously.
8. If you don't get any answers today, ask if you can come tomorrow.
9. Do this for ten to fifteen minutes, every day for one week.
10. Keep remembering that your friend must have confidence in you.
11. Your friend has power and can resolve problems, so pay close attention.
12. If your friend doesn't appear, don't panic. A friend will often appear only at stress times, when needed most.

Index

Acupuncture, 30–31
Aeltzer, Arnold, 17
Agassiz, Louis, 25
American Psychological Association, 133
American Society of Clinical Hypnosis, 28–29
American University, 16
Amoeba and evolution, 37
Anders, Thomas, 74
Andhra Research University of India, 22
Asimov, Isaac, 91
Automatic nervous system, 54
Awareness exercises, 33–34, 48–49, 61–62, 83–84, 103–105, 128
Axons, 55
Beecher, H.K., 107
Berkshire Music Center, 117
Billion Dollar Brain, The, 36
Bleier, Robert "Rocky," 115–116
Bloom, Molly, 70
Body thermostat, 44
Boylan Blazes, 70
Brain
- appearance, 41–42
- cerebellum, 43
- cerebral hemispheres, 42
- cortex, 40, 64
- development, 39–40
- hemispheres, 46–47
- major parts of, 43–46
- medulla, 49
- nervous systems, 54, 58–59

pons, 49
potential, 26
power, 15
reticular activating system, 50
search brain, 38
size, 40
smell brain, 38
stem, 49
uniqueness, 19
universal network, 21
visual brain, 38
Brandeis University, 133
Bressler, David, 139
Brooklyn College, 133
Brown, Kingdon L., 22
Buckley, William F., 84
Bucy, Paul, 46
Bulgarian Rapid-Learning Method, 136–137

Caduceus emblem, 76
Cancer Counseling and Research Center (Fort Worth), 124–127
Carnival of the Animals, 49
Cerebellum, 43, 63
Cerebral hemispheres, 42
Cerebrum, 45, 50, 63
Chagall, Marc, 78
Chardin, Tielhard de, 135
Child Buyer, The, 35
Churchill, Winston, 96
Cirlot, J. E., 76
Columbia University, 109
Complex reflexes, 56
Copland, Aaron, 116
Cortex, 40–41, 45–46, 64
Coué, Emile, 119
Creighton, James, 127
Cybernetics, 113
Dali symbolism, 78
Dedalus, Stephen, 70
Deighton, Len, 26
Dement, William, 73
Dendrites, 55
Devi, Shakuntula, 16
Dictionary of Symbols, A, 76
Diederich, Paul, 69
Dukas, Paul, 49
Duke University, 24

Ebbinghaus, Hermann, 95
Eccles, Sir John, 137
Edison, Thomas Alva, 23, 118
Educational Testing Service, 69
Eliot, Alexander, 71–72
Embryonic development, 40
Emerson, Ralph Waldo, 24
Engrams, 90
Endorphins, 30, 108
ESB (electrical stimulation of the brain), 19–20
ESP (extrasensory perception), 23
Exercises to relax, 59–60, 62

Felsen, Richard, 108
Fields, Howard L., 108
Forebrain, 43–44, 51–52, 67–68
Frost, Robert, 77
Fuller, R. Buckminster, 123

Ganglions, 38
Gardner, John W., 132
Gallwey, W. Timothy, 115
Geller, Uri, 123
George Mason Community College, 16

Georgetown University, 17, 107
George Washington University, 16
Getting Well Again, 127

Harris, Mark G., 113
Harvard University, 107
Hemispheres of the brain, 46–47
Hersey, John, 35
Hindbrain, 43–44, 51–52
Holistic health, 122–125
Holmes, Oliver Wendell, 128
Hook words as memory aids, 99
Hugo, Victor, 92
Human Brain, The, 51
Human Engineering Laboratories, 68
Hyden, Holger, 90
Hypnotism, 28–30
  as a control, 29
  as memory aid, 29
  as posthypnotic suggestion, 30
Hypothalamus, 44, 50, 64

Images and the brain, 67, 71–75
Inner Game of Tennis, The, 115
Institute of Suggestology, 136
Irwin Army Hospital, 116

James, William, 31, 92
Joyce, James, 70
Jung, Carl G., 74

Kandinsky, Wassily, 78
Katz, Ronald, 30
Klee, Paul, 78
Kleitman, Nathaniel, 73

Language, 67–68
Lear, Bill, 53
Lecky, Prescott, 109
Le Corbusier, 77
Lehmann College, 137
Lieberman, Alex, 78
Lorayne, Harry, 88
Lozanov, Georgi, 135–136
Lucas, Jerry, 88
Luria, A. R., 94

Maslow, Abraham H., 133
Massachusetts General Hospital, 29
Mathews-Simonton, Stephanie, 127
Mead, Margaret, 31
Medical School of Virginia, 31
Medulla, 49
Memory, 87–97
  association, 100
  hook words, 99
  improving and expanding, 85–97
  linking, 99
  numbers, 102
  phases, 90
  variables, 93
Memory Book, The, 88
Mentalists, 97–98
Metempsychosis, 70
Michaelangelo, 25, 66–67
Midbrain, 43–44, 51
Milton, John, 92
Mind Can Do Anything, The, 123
Mind of a Mnemonist, The, 94
M.I.T. (Massachusetts Institute of Technology), 113
Mnemonists, 98–99
Montreal Neurological Institute, 19
Moore, Henry, 78
Motherwell, Robert, 118
Motor nerve cells, 54, 64

Mrs. Dalloway, 79–80
Mulligan, Buck, 70
Murphy, Joseph, 22
Mussorgsky, Modest Petrovich, 49

Napoleon, 96
National Institute of Mental Health, 30
Neanderthal man, 63
Nervous system, 54, 57–58
Neuron cells, 54–55
New Angles on Putting, 114
Nicklaus, Jack, 117
Notre Dame Cathedral, 77
Northwestern University, 46

O'Connor, Johnson, 68–69
Oriental detachment exercise, 62
O'Shea, John "Pat," 117
Ostrander, Nancy, 135
Ostrander, Sheila, 135
Oyle, Irving, 123–124, 139

Paradise Lost, 92
Pavlov, Ivan, 107
Penfield, Wilder, 19
Peptide proteins, 30
Pert, Agu, 30
Peripheral nervous system, 54
Pfeiffer, John, 51
Picasso, Pablo, 72
Pictures at an Exhibition, 49
Pittsburgh Steelers, 116
Pollack, Cecilia, 137
Pons, 49
Power of Psychic Awareness, The, 22
Psychic experiences, 21–23
Psychic Perception: The Magic of Extrasensory Power, 23
Psychology Today, 108

Ramey, Estelle, 107
Receptor cells, 17
Reflexes, 56
Relaxing exercises, 59–60, 62
REM (rapid eye movement), 73
Reticular Activating System, 50, 64
Rhine, J.B., 23
Rite of Spring, The, 49
RNA (ribonucleic acid), 90–91
Roberts, Dirk, 69–70
Roffwarg, Howard, 74
Ross, Thelma, 123

Saint-Saëns, Charles Camille, 49
Sands Point Country Day School, 31–32
Satyr, 92
Saving the Queen, 84
Savoye House (France), 77
Schroeder, Lynn, 135
Schubert, Franz Peter, 24–25
Search brain, 38
Self-Renewal, 132
Sensory nerve cells, 54, 64
Shealy, C. Norman, 122
Sight and Insight, 71–72
Simenon, Georges, 108
Simonton, O. Carl, 124–127, 139
Simple reflexes, 56
Smelch, George, 108
Smell brain, 38
Sorcerer's Apprentice, The, 49
Spiegel, David, 29–30
Spinal cord, 49, 54, 56
Stained Glass, 84

Stanford University Medical School, 73–74
State University of New York at Albany, 108
Stem of brain, 49, 56
"Stopping by Woods on a Snowy Evening," 77
Stravinsky, Igor, 49
Saint Timothy's Abbey Church (Detroit), 22
Suggestology theory, 136
Super Learning, 135
Sword in the Stone, The, 63
Symbols, 67, 75–78

Thinkies (daily experiments), 34–36, 62–63, 84–86
Thalamus, 44–45, 50, 63
Thermostat of the body, 44
Time, 71
Travis Air Force Base, 124

UCLA Medical School Pain Center, 122, 139
Ulene, Art, 139
Ulysses, 70
University College (Dublin), 108
University of California at Los Angeles, 30
University of California, San Francisco, 107
University of California, Santa Cruz, 123
University of Goteborg (Sweden), 90
University of Moscow, 94
University of Oregon Medical School, 124
University of Texas Health Sciences Center, 74
University of Toronto, 30
University of Washington, 31
USAF Medical Center, 126

Vocabulary Builder, 69
Vogt, Andy, 17
Voluntary nervous system, 54

Walter, W. Grey, 15
Wesley Hospital, 46
White, T.H., 63
Whitman, Thomas Bay, 27–28
Who's Afraid of Virginia Woolf?, 79
Wiener, Norbert, 113
Winston, Peter, 31–32
Woolf, Virginia, 78–80
Worrell, Olga, 123